Biosensors for Tackling Antimicrobial Resistance (AMR)

Vishal Chaudhary • Nikhil Bhalla
Editors

Biosensors for Tackling Antimicrobial Resistance (AMR)

Combating Antibiotic Abuse

Springer

Editors
Vishal Chaudhary
Nakhonsawan Studiorum
for Advanced Studies
Centre for Theoretical Physics and Natural
Philosophy, Mahidol University
Phayuha Khiri, Nakhon Sawan, Thailand

Nikhil Bhalla
Nanotechnology and Integrated
Bioengineering Centre (NIBEC)
School of Engineering
Ulster University
Belfast, United Kingdom

ISBN 978-981-95-9150-3 ISBN 978-981-95-9151-0 (eBook)
https://doi.org/10.1007/978-981-95-9151-0

This Springer imprint is published by the registered company Springer Nature Singapore Pte Ltd.
The registered company address is: 152 Beach Road, #21-01/04 Gateway East, Singapore 189721, Singapore

Dr. Vishal Chaudhary dedicates this book to the memory of his father Late Chaudhary Rajkumar Kadian. Dr Nikhil Bhalla dedicates this book to the memory of his grandmother, Ram Dei Bhalla

Foreword

The urgency of the Antimicrobial Resistance (AMR) crisis cannot be overstated, as it is silently creating a pandemic situation. We are at a critical point in time where the speed of microbial evolution is outpacing the development of new drugs, which is overwhelming our current healthcare facilities. What is clear is that simply developing new antibiotics is insufficient, as it is time-consuming; we must also master the art of effective surveillance and control over antibiotic misuse, following the phrase that "prevention is better than cure".

This timely volume addresses exactly this need in the context of the One Health. The authors have expertly framed a work that moves from the foundational understanding of antibiotic abuse to the sophisticated integration of biosensors within holistic surveillance systems to avert AMR. By integrating cutting-edge technologies like artificial intelligence, bioinformatics, and the unique geographical insights offered by geospatial analysis, the book provides a strong roadmap for the future of One Health monitoring.

It is rare to find a book that so effectively combines the molecular science of detection with the macroscopic strategy of surveillance. This is not merely a collection of research, but it is a call to action and a toolkit for scientists, engineers, and policymakers. I highly recommend this book as an essential resource for anyone serious about tackling the AMR challenge head-on.

Professor of Advanced Materials
School of Engineering
Ulster University
Belfast, United Kingdom

Pagona Papakonstantinou
p.papakonstantinou@ulster.ac.uk

Preface

The global rise of Antimicrobial Resistance (AMR) stands as one of the most pressing One Health challenges of the present time. It is significantly fuelled by the massive misuse and abuse of antibiotics. This crisis overwhelms the present healthcare system and threatens the decades of medical progress, potentially turning common infections untreatable.

This book aims to bridge the critical gap between understanding the medical and environmental roots of the AMR crisis and deploying cutting-edge technological solutions in the form of biosensors for effective surveillance and control. Starting with a fundamental outlook at the problem, we delve into innovative monitoring techniques like wastewater surveillance before focusing on the core solution: the next generation of biosensors.

We offer a comprehensive exploration of biosensors, their components, features, and practical applications, detailing case studies on diversified, i.e., electrical/electrochemical and optical, biosensors specifically designed for antibiotic abuse detection. Furthermore, we examine the future of surveillance through the integration of artificial intelligence, machine learning, bioinformatics, and geospatial analysis into robust surveillance systems to avert AMR. Finally, a practical tutorial is included to guide readers in developing simple biosensors.

This volume is intended for researchers, engineers, physicists, clinicians, public health officials, and advanced students committed to fighting AMR. It is our hope that the insights and tools presented within these chapters will inspire the next generation of solutions needed to safeguard global health against this silent pandemic.

Phayuha Khiri, Nakhon Sawan, Thailand — Vishal Chaudhary
Belfast, UK — Nikhil Bhalla

Acknowledgements

We owe a profound debt of gratitude to the many individuals and organisations who contributed, directly and indirectly, to the completion of this book.

First and foremost, we extend our sincere thanks to the authors and contributors for their expertise, dedication, and tireless efforts in changing complex research into accessible and understandable chapters. The depth of knowledge and spanning medical perspectives to biosensor technology, along with geospatial analysis, is a testament to your collaborative spirit to fight the silent pandemic of AMR.

We are grateful to Springer for their support and guidance throughout the publication process.

To our respective families and friends, thank you for your patience, understanding, and unwavering support during the countless hours spent researching and writing. Vishal edited this book in the memory of his father, Late Chaudhary Rajkumar Kadian and Nikhil edited this book in the memory of his grandmother, Ram Dei Bhalla.

Vishal and Nikhil are also thankful to the British Council for providing us funding under its Going Global program with collaboration of Industry-Academia to solve the global problem of AMR by detecting antibiotic abuse and avert the first stage of this cause. Through this initiative, Vishal and Nikhil developed forged a collaboration on AMR that culminated in the development of a dedicated course on AMR, with some key insights and notes captured in this book.

We extend our thanks to the respective universities, i.e., Ulster University and Mahidol University, for unwavering support. Vishal also wishes to extend thanks to his previous institution the University of Delhi, India, which helped him to lay the foundation of this work. He also wishes to sincerely thank Prof. Burin Gumjudpai, Founding Director and Professor of Theoretical Physics at the Centre for Theoretical Physics & Natural Philosophy "Nakhonsawan Studiorum for Advanced Studies", Mahidol University, Nakhonsawan Campus, for continuous support and motivation.

Finally, we acknowledge the global scientific community, including the researchers and innovators whose foundational work in microbiology, analytical chemistry, physics and One Health has paved the way for the development of the surveillance technologies discussed herein.

Contents

Editors and Contributors

About the Editors

Vishal Chaudhary is Lecturer of Physics of Complex Life-Matter Interface Dynamics and Sensor Intelligence at Centre for Theoretical Physics and Natural Philosophy, Nakhonsawan Studiorum for Advanced Studies, Nakhonsawan Campus, Mahidol University, Thailand, since April 2025. Prior to this, he served as Assistant Professor of Physics at the University of Delhi, India, for 8 years. He obtained his BSc (H) in Physics First Class, and MSc and PhD in Physics from the University of Delhi, India. He has been associated with the development of sensors, including gas sensors, biosensors, and nanosensors, which integrate modern-day technology, including, nanotechnology, artificial intelligence, bioinformatics, and medical diagnostics for One Health management, raising the era of Sensor Intelligence and green semiconductors as pioneer. He is well recognised for his contributions to sensors, complex physics and nanotechnology-based One Health Management, attested by over 160 research publications in journals of international repute. He has been honoured with several recognitions, including the Agents of Change Award 2023, Top 2% Scientists World 2023, 2024 and 2025, Associate Editor at ECS Sensor Plus and Sceintific Reports, SDG Service Award 2021, and Silver Country Coordinator Award 2022, for research and society contributions, with emphasis on LGBTQIA+ Community.

Nikhil Bhalla is currently working as an Assistant Professor in the University of Ulster, UK. His research is in the area of biosensing with a prime focus on nanoplasmonic technologies and interfacial science of biosensing materials, transducers, and biorecognition layers. He focuses on the use of his developed sensors for healthcare and food applications. He did his postdoctoral training at OIST, Japan, with Professor Amy Shen after receiving his PhD from the University of Bath, UK, in 2016, MS in Microelectronics and Applications from CYCU, Taiwan, and a first division honours degree (B.E. Hons) in Electronics and Instrumentation Engineering from BITS-Pilani, India.

Contributors

Ali J. Addie Center of Industrial Applications and Materials Technology, Scientific Research Commission, Baghdad, Iraq

Moses Sunday Afariogun Department of Cell Biology and Genetics, University of Lagos, Akoka, Nigeria

Safeer Ahmed Department of Chemistry, Quaid-I-Azam University, Islamabad, Pakistan

Muafia Akbar Department of Chemistry, University of Okara, Okara, Pakistan

Norhana Arsad Photonics Technology Lab, Department of Electrical, Electronic and Systems Engineering, Faculty of Engineering and Built Environment, Universiti Kebangsaan Malaysia, UKM, Bangi, Malaysia

Aagam L. Bamb Biochemical Science Division, National Chemical Laboratory, Pune, India

Stefania Bertazzon University of Calgary, Calgary, AB, Canada

O'Brien Institute for Public Health, Calgary, AB, Canada

Nikhil Bhalla Nanotechnology and Integrated Bioengineering Centre (NIBEC), School of Engineering, Ulster University, Belfast, Northern Ireland, UK

Eshi Bhutani Atal Bihari Vajpayee Institute of Medical Sciences and Dr. Ram Manohar Lohia Hospital, New Delhi, India

Akshay Chawla School of Advanced Chemical Sciences, Shoolini University, Solan, HP, India

Pankaj Gautam Department of Microbiology, Graphic Era (Deemed to be University), Dehradun, Uttarakhand, India

Adawiya J. Haider Applied Sciences Department/Laser Science and Technology Branch, University of Technology, Baghdad, Iraq

Sarvesh B. Jadhav SoilSens Pvt. Ltd., Pune, India

Zul Kamal Chongqing University of Chinese Medicines, Chongqing, People's Republic of China

Shaheed Benazir Bhutto University, Sheringal, Khyber Pakhtunkhwa, Pakistan

Ajita Kapur Department of Pharmacology, Atal Bihari Vajpayee Institute of Medical Sciences and Dr. Ram Manohar Lohia Hospital, New Delhi, India

Kashif Ali Khan Chongqing University of Chinese Medicines, Chongqing, People's Republic of China

Navin Kumar Department of Biotechnology, Graphic Era (Deemed to be University), Dehradun, Uttarakhand, India

Rahul Kumar Department of Microbiology, Graphic Era (Deemed to be University), Dehradun, Uttarakhand, India

Ayush Madan Department of Biotechnology, School of Research and Technology, People's University, Bhopal, Madhya Pradesh, India

Stephen Olaosebikan Makanjuola Department of Medical Laboratory Science, Faculty of Allied Health Science, Elizade University, Ilara-Mokin, Nigeria

Debasis Mitra Department of Microbiology, Graphic Era (Deemed to be University), Dehradun, Uttarakhand, India

Ghulam Mustafa Department of Chemistry, University of Okara, Okara, Pakistan

Mahesh Narayan Department of Chemistry and Biochemistry, The University of Texas at El Paso, El Paso, TX, USA

Abosede Olubunmi Obadina Department of Public Health, College of Allied Health Science, McPherson University, Seriki Sotayo, Nigeria

Ismail Babatunde Onajobi Department of Microbiology, Faculty of Science, Olabisi Onabanjo University, Ago-Iwoye, Nigeria

Diksha Pathania Dairy Technology Division, National Dairy Research Institute (ICAR), Karnal, Haryana, India

Aashi Sable University of Kassel, Witzenhausen, Germany

Hochschule Fulda, University of Applied Sciences, Fulda, Germany

Harsh Sable Department of Forensic Science, School of Life and Applied Sciences, Maya Devi University, Dehradun, Uttarakhand, India

Nauman Sadiq Department of Chemistry, Quaid-I-Azam University, Islamabad, Pakistan

Department of Chemistry, University of Okara, Okara, Pakistan

Oyindamola John Samson Department of Microbiology, Faculty of Science, Olabisi Onabanjo University, Ago-Iwoye, Nigeria

Department of Microbiology and Biotechnology, Faculty of Natural Sciences, Ajayi Crowther University, Oyo, Nigeria

Muhammad Shafiq Research Institute of Clinical Pharmacy, Department of Pharmacology, Shantou University Medical College, Guangdong, China

Rizwan Shahid University of Calgary, Calgary, AB, Canada

O'Brien Institute for Public Health, Calgary, AB, Canada

Primary Care Alberta, Calgary, AB, Canada

Sadaf Shaikh Syngene International Limited, Hyderabad, India

Pardeep Singh School of Advanced Chemical Sciences, Shoolini University, Solan, HP, India

Vandana Singh Department of Microbiology, Sharda School of Allied Health Sciences, Sharda University, Greater Noida, UP, India

Vedashree Sirdeshmukh Defence Institute of Advanced Technology, Pune, India

Vatika Soni School of Advanced Chemical Sciences, Shoolini University, Solan, HP, India

Sonu Sonu School of Advanced Chemical Sciences, Shoolini University, Solan, HP, India

Chandrakant Tagad Department of Biochemistry, SBES College, S.B.E.S. College of Science, Chhatrapati Sambhajinagar (Aurangabad), Maharashtra, India

Bakr Ahmed Taha Photonics Technology Lab, Department of Electrical, Electronic and Systems Engineering, Faculty of Engineering and Built Environment, Universiti Kebangsaan Malaysia, UKM, Bangi, Malaysia

Al-imam University College, Balad, Iraq

Bashir Ullah Chongqing University of Chinese Medicines, Chongqing, People's Republic of China

Muhammad Usman Department of Electronics, Quaid-I-Azam University, Islamabad, Pakistan

Tanja Vasić Faculty of Agriculture, University of Niš, Kruševac, Serbia

Sumedh Yewale University of Michigan, Ann Arbor, MI, USA

Understanding Antibiotics: Medical Perspectives 1

Ajita Kapur and Eshi Bhutani

1.1 Introduction

Antimicrobials are one of the most significant achievements of modern medicine. Their use has revolutionized the treatment of a wide miscellany of fatal infectious diseases and dramatically improved patient outcomes and increased life expectancy across the globe.

The specific and diverse nature of antimicrobials is against a wide spectrum of pathogenic mechanisms by which the microbes produce disease. They have increased activity for targets that are unique to prokaryotes, fungi or viruses. The target can be to inhibit cell wall synthesis, inhibit bacterial ribosomes or the DNA replication and propagation mechanisms, or to damage the DNA. A myriad of other mechanisms exist within the functions of antimicrobial agents with different complexities and specialities, but these can be grouped broadly as covered in this chapter.

Antibiotics were originally substances produced by microorganisms, which restricted the growth of, or killed other microorganisms. The different classes of antibiotics were discovered to be natural products of fungi, bacteria, and actinomycetes. They were extracted, purified and concentrated for their use as therapeutic agents in humans. New antibiotics consisted of semisynthetic and synthetic derivatives of the same.

A. Kapur (✉)
Department of Pharmacology, Atal Bihari Vajpayee Institute of Medical Sciences and Dr. Ram Manohar Lohia Hospital, New Delhi, India

E. Bhutani
Atal Bihari Vajpayee Institute of Medical Sciences and Dr. Ram Manohar Lohia Hospital, New Delhi, India

V. Chaudhary, N. Bhalla (eds.), *Biosensors for Tackling Antimicrobial Resistance (AMR)*, https://doi.org/10.1007/978-981-95-9151-0_1

The term antimicrobial agents includes both naturally derived drugs as well as the synthetic agents. Pharmacophore refers to the active chemical moiety of the antimicrobial drug.

Antimicrobial molecules can be seen as ligands whose receptors are microbial proteins. The receptors they bind to, and interrupt, are essential in the biochemical pathways of the microbes and interfere with their structure and physiology.

The major problem threatening the continued success of antimicrobials is the development of antimicrobial resistance (AMR). According to a UN report, drug-resistant diseases could cause 10 million deaths each year by 2050 and damage to the economy as catastrophic as during the 2008–2009 global financial crisis. By 2030, antimicrobial resistance could force up to 24 million people into extreme poverty [1].

1.2 Classification of Antibiotics

Broadly, antimicrobials can be classified on the basis of the main categories of microorganisms they are effective against i.e. antibacterial, antifungal, antiviral and antiparasitic agents. However, some agents work against more than one category of microorganisms. Further, these can be grouped under the following headings.

1. Based on the chemical structure of its pharmacophore.
2. Based on the spectrum of action.
3. Based on the biochemical pathway interfered

1.2.1 Classification Based on Chemical Structure

The different families of antimicrobials have various members and each presents a unique chemical structure, which is associated with its distinctive behaviour with respect to its reactions with microbes. On this basis, antibiotics can be categorized into the classes included in Table 1.1 [2]. Cephalosporins belonging to the beta lactam group of antibiotics can be further divided into five generations based on the spectrum and their temporal discovery (Table 1.2) (Fig. 1.1).

1.2.2 Classification Based on Spectrum of Action

This classification divides antibiotics into narrow spectrum and broad spectrum based on the range of effects (Table 1.3).

The narrow spectrum antibiotics were typically the ones used against specific microorganisms, whereas the broad-spectrum antibiotics are used when the specific organism causing the disease is not known, so these provide protection against a wider range.

Table 1.1 Classification of antibiotics based on chemical structure

Antibiotic class	Class structure	Examples
Aminoglycosides	Characterised by a core structure of amino sugars connected via glycosidic linkages to a dibasic aminocyclitol. They are polycationic and their polarity is partly responsible for their pharmacokinetic properties [3]	Gentamicin, tobramycin, amikacin, kanamycin, streptomycin and neomycin. Neoglycoside: Plazomicin
Beta lactams	All members share the beta lactam ring as the essential core structure, and most have an additional structure directly attached to the beta lactam ring, except for monobactams [4]	Penicillins: Penicillin G, penicillin V, methicillin, ampicillin, amoxicillin, piperacillin, temocillin Cephalosporins: Distributed in five generations (Table 1.2) [5] Siderophore cephalosporin: Cefiderocol Carbapenems: Imipenem, ertapenem, meropenem and doripenem Monobactams (monocyclic beta lactam): Aztreonam
Diaminopyrimidines	Organic antibiotics having a pyrimidine ring substituted by two amine groups [6]	Trimethoprim and pyrimethamine
Glycopeptides	They are glycoside cyclic or polycyclic peptides [7]	Vancomycin, bacitracin and teicoplanin
Lincosamides	These consist of amino acid l-proline linked to lincosamine via amide bond	Clindamycin and lincomycin
Lipopeptides	Usually contain macrocyclic peptide cores with a hydrocarbon tail, and are negatively charged	Daptomycin
Macrolides and Ketolides	They are macrocyclic compounds containing a macro lactone ring, usually having 14 to 16 atoms substituted by bipolar and nonpolar groups and linked to one or more sugars glycosidic bonds [8] Ketolides are structurally similar to macrolides but have a 3-keto group substituent	Macrolides: Erythromycin and its semisynthetic derivatives like clarithromycin and azithromycin Ketolides: Telithromycin
Nicotinic acid derivatives	These are polymorphs (may exist in more than one crystal form) derived from nicotinic acid	Isoniazid, ethionamide and pyrazinamide
Nitroimidazoles	These are C-nitro compounds [9]	Metronidazole and tinidazole
Oxazolidinones	Synthetic organofluorine compounds [10]	Linezolid and tedizolid
Phenicols	Organochlorine compounds containing a nitrobenzene ring [11]	Chloramphenicol

(continued)

Table 1.1 (continued)

Antibiotic class	Class structure	Examples
Quinolones	Synthetic antibacterials consisting of a bicyclic ring. The addition of a fluorine atom at position C6 and substitutions on the basic quinolone structure yield different agents known as fluoroquinolones [12–14]	Nalidixic acid, ciprofloxacin, norfloxacin, ofloxacin, levofloxacin
Streptogramins	Streptogramins consist of two different molecules, the group A streptogramins, which are polyunsaturated macrolactones,	Quinupristin/Dalfopristin is a two-drug combination of two semisynthetic derivatives [15]
	And the group B streptogramins, which are cyclic hexadepsipeptides [16]	
Sulfonamides	Organosulphur compounds characterised by the existence of sulfanilamide group and a distinct six or five membered heterocyclic ring [17, 18]	Sulfamethoxazole, sulfamethizole, sulfamerazine, sulfisoxazole and sulfasalazine
Tetracyclines and Glycylcyclines	Tetracyclines consist of a linear fused tetracyclic nucleus to which a variety of functional groups are attached [19]. Glycylcyclines are synthetic tetracycline analogues. Fluorocycline are synthetic tetracycline with fluorine substitution	Tetracyclines: Chlortetracycline, oxytetracycline, doxycycline, and minocycline Glycylcyclines: Tigecycline Fluorocycline: Eravacycline

Table 1.2 Cephalosporins grouped into 5 different generations [5]

Classification of Cephalosporins	Common drugs in use
First generation	Cefazolin, cephalexin
Second generation	Cefuroxime, Cefprozil
Third generation	Ceftriaxone, Cefoperazone, Ceftazidime
Fourth generation	Cefepime, Cefpirome
Fifth generation	Ceftaroline, Ceftobiprole

However, this polar classification is often misapplied and overly ambiguous. Although the broad-spectrum antibiotics suggest a greater therapeutic reliability, especially in cases of empirical therapy where the exact bacteria are unknown; this categorisation does not always reflect the reality of bacterial resistance.

Additionally, narrow spectrum antibiotics are thought to be more effective in preventing resistance, but this is not always the case. In fact, some bacteria are naturally resistant to narrow spectrum antibiotics, and the emergence of resistance otherwise is much more complex than being linked to the spectrum of activity.

Rather than labelling different drugs as narrow or broad spectrum, it would be better to differentiate them on the basis of specific bacteria involved, their clinical indicators and the resistance patterns for better treatment outcomes [20–22].

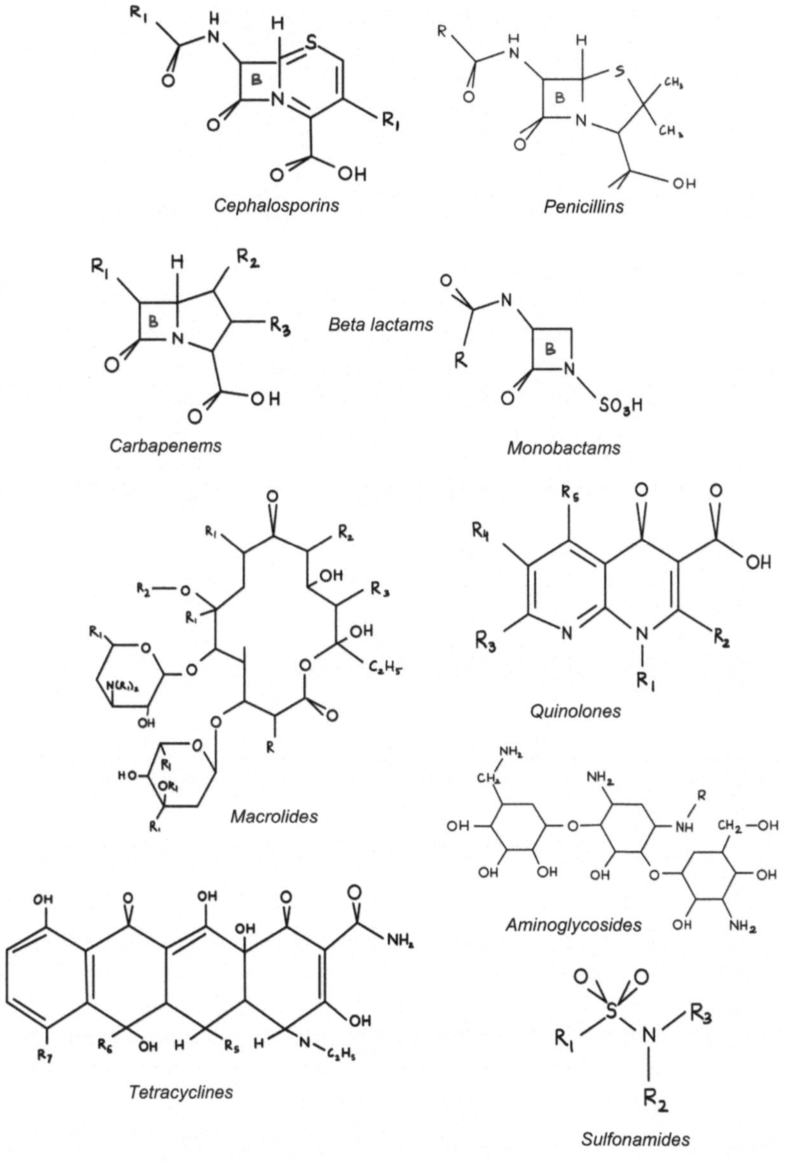

Fig. 1.1 Structures of common antibiotics

1.2.3 Classification Based on Mechanism of Action

The final classification discussed here is based on the different mechanisms of action shown by various antibiotic classes (Table 1.4) [7, 23–25].

Table 1.3 Antibiotic classes grouped according to their spectrum of activity

Narrow Spectrum Antibiotics	1st and second generation cephalosporins Narrow spectrum penicillins Aztreonam Colistins Daptomycin
Broad Spectrum antibiotics	3rd and fourth generation cephalosporins macrolides Chloramphenicol Broad spectrum penicillins quinolones

1.3 Uses of Antibiotics

Antibiotics are widely in use all across the globe, in institutional as well as domestic spheres. They are one of the most frequently prescribed drugs across all divisions. They work by either killing or inhibiting the growth of bacteria.

The most important use of antibiotics is the treatment of bacterial infections ranging from mild infections to grievous diseases. These infections can affect all systems of the body and commonly include but are not limited to the following:

- Respiratory tract infections
- Urinary tract infections
- Soft tissue and skin infections
- Brain infections
- Gastrointestinal tract and abdominal infections
- Sexually transmitted diseases

The treatment given for these infections can be empirical without the definitive identification of specific causative organisms. This constitutes currently the most common clinical use.

Definitive therapy is instituted after the identification of organisms and the susceptibility results.

Antibiotics are also used prophylactically for the prevention of bacterial infections. The prophylaxis can be primary prophylaxis which involves administering antibiotics to individuals who are not yet infected. Preemptive therapy is given to infected individuals before the appearance of signs and symptoms of diseases. Sometimes the secondary or suppressive prophylaxis is continued beyond the treatment example among the immunocompromised host. The common conditions where antimicrobial prophylaxis is given includes:

- **Surgical prophylaxis for surgical site infections (SSI)**

The purpose of surgical prophylaxis is to reduce the incidence of SSI like superficial incisional infections, deep incisional infections and organ or space infections; with little to no changes in the host microbial flora.

Table 1.4 Various antibiotics and their classes grouped on the basis of their mechanism of action

Mechanism of action		Antibiotic class		Antibiotics	
Cell Wall Synthesis inhibitors		Beta lactams	Penicillins	Penicillin G, penicillin V, methicillin, ampicillin, amoxicillin, piperacillin	
			Cephalosporins	First generation	Cefazolin, cephalexin
				Second generation	Cefuroxime, Cefprozil
				Third generation	Ceftriaxone, Cefoperazone, Ceftazidime
				Fourth generation	Cefepime
				Fifth generation	Ceftaroline, Ceftobiprole
			Carbapenems	Imipenem, Ertapenem, Meropenem	
			Monobactams	Aztreonam	
		Glycopeptides		Vancomycin, bacitracin, Teicoplanin, Polymyxin B	
Protein synthesis inhibitors	30S	Tetracyclines		Chlortetracycline, Oxytetracycline, doxycycline, minocycline, Eravacycline	
		Aminoglycosides[a]		Gentamicin, tobramycin, amikacin, kanamycin, streptomycin, neomycin, Plazomicin[b]	
	50S	Macrolides		Erythromycins, azithromycin, clarithromycin	
		Oxazolidinones		Linezolid	
		Streptogramins		Quinupristin/Dalfopristin	
		Lincosamides		Clindamycin, Lincomycin	
				Chloramphenicol	
Inhibition of DNA topoisomerases		Quinolones		Nalidixic acid, ciprofloxacin, Norfloxacin, Ofloxacin, levofloxacin	
Inhibition of folic acid synthesis		Sulfonamides		Sulfamethoxazole, Sulfamethizole, Sulfamerazine, Sulfisoxazole, sulfasalazine	
		DHFR[c] inhibitors		Trimethoprim	
Cause DNA damage		Nitroimidazoles		Metronidazole, Tinidazole	
Inhibit mRNA synthesis				Rifampicin	

[a]*Aminoglycosides, along with working as protein synthesis inhibitors by attaching to the 30S subunit and additional sites on the 50S subunit and even to the 30S–50S interface, have an additional action of causing misreading of DNA, which affects the permeability of the sensitive bacteria. This allows ions, amino acids, and even proteins to leak out leading to cell death*

[b]*Plazomicin is a newer aminoglycoside with rationally designed semi-synthetic structure, often classified as neoglycoside*

[c]*Dihydrofolate reductase*

- **Prevention of infections in immunocompromised patients**
  Long-term antimicrobial prophylaxis is recommended in immunocompromised patients to prevent infections such as Pneumocyctis jiroveci pneumonia (PJP), toxoplasmosis, nocardiosis etc. Bactericidal, inexpensive antibiotics having low toxicity profile and minimal drug-drug interactions should be preferred. For example, cotrimoxazole is preferred for prophylaxis against PJP [2, 26–31].

- **Post exposure prophylaxis**
  This form of prophylaxis is extremely important in preventing disease in patients who have been exposed to the risk factor, and reduces morbidity and mortality. This is commonly used for preventing sexually transmitted infections (example after needle stick injury) and respiratory infections.

- **Pre Exposure Prophylaxis**
  This is a lesser practiced form of prophylaxis which is used in preventing infections in high-risk situations; for contacts of patients with diseases which have high mortality (example those who are sexual partners with HIV) or during epidemics.

- **Prevention of specific diseases, like Infective endocarditis**
  Antibiotic prophylaxis against Streptococcus viridans is given during high risk invasive oral, dental, gastrourinary and gastrointestinal procedures to prevent infective endocarditis.

1.4 Selection of Antibiotics

The selection of appropriate antimicrobial agents depends upon the infecting microorganisms, site of infection and the type of patient to be treated. As far as possible, the choice of antibiotic should be based on identification of microorganism and its susceptibility pattern.

Diffusion tests using disks impregnated with antimicrobial drugs can be used for testing susceptibility patterns of bacteria. The bacteria from the sample are plated on a solid growth.

medium and incubated for 12 to 24 hours. Based on the size of the area without the bacterial growth around each disk (called the zone of inhibition) the isolate is categorized as resistant, intermediate susceptible or susceptible. In Dilution tests, the antibiotics are used in serial dilutions in a liquid broth medium (Mueller–Hinton (MH) medium) in which a culture of the test microorganism is added. **Minimum inhibitory concentration** (MIC) refers to the lowest in vitro concentration of the antibacterial drug (in mg/L) that prevents visible growth of an organism completely. The MIC for each drug is compared to the breakpoints established for that antibiotic-microorganism pair. The isolate is considered susceptible when the MIC is at or below the breakpoint for that antibiotic-microorganism pair. If the microorganisms are placed in a medium without antibiotics after exposure of an antibiotic media then they start multiplying again after a lag period. This time required for resumption of growth of bacteria is called the **post-antibiotic effect**. A dose-dependent long post- antibiotic effect is shown by aminoglycosides, fluoroquinolones and rifampicin [32–36].

Minimum bactericidal concentration (MBC) is the concentration of an antibiotic that kills the majority of bacteria (99.9%). MBC is estimated by subculturing from the dilution test tubes with no visible growth in an antibiotic free media. If the growth reappears then the bacteria were only inhibited in dilution test whereas no growth depicts bacterial killing. A small difference in MBC and MIC depicts the bactericidal nature of the antibiotic. Bactericidal antibiotics are in general preferred more in cases of severe infections and in immunocompromised patients.

Empirical therapy has to be initiated only in cases of severe infections after obtaining samples for culture and drug susceptibility testing. Patient factors such as age, renal and hepatic functions, pregnancy, immune status, allergy status and genetic factors should also be considered for choosing the appropriate antibiotic. Antibiotics to be avoided in particular patient populations are included in Table 1.5.

A crucial consideration for selecting an antimicrobial for therapy is the site of the infection. The antimicrobial should be able to penetrate the anatomical compartment which indeed depends upon the chemical nature of the drug and presence of multidrug transporters. Production of biofilms by bacteria causing chronic recurrent infections such as in patients of cystic fibrosis, chronic osteomyelitis and in patients with prosthetic devices such as indwelling catheters, artificial heart valves etc. can act as barriers to penetration of the drug. Selection of antimicrobial agents should also be based on whether it belongs to Access, Watch or Reserve groups as per WHO AWaRe classification. The antimicrobials belonging to the Access and Watch group have lower potential for resistance and should be preferred for common infections whereas those belonging to the Reserve group (such as linezolid, colistin and polymyxin) should be used only as last option against multidrug resistant organisms [31, 37, 38].

Table 1.5 Common antibiotics to be avoided in particular patient populations

Paediatric population	Pregnancy	Hepatic diseases	Renal diseases
Chloramphenicol Tetracycline Fluoroquinolones	Tetracycline Cotrimoxazole Fluoroquinolones Chloramphenicol Sulfonamides Nitrofurantoin	Tetracycline Erythromycin Pyrazinamide Nalidixic Acid Chloramphenicol Isoniazid Metronidazole Rifampicin Clindamycin	Nalidixic Acid Tetracycline Nitrofurantoin Amphotericin B Aminoglycosides Ethambutol Vancomycin

1.5 Selection of Dosing Schedule

Selection of the dosing schedule depends on the MIC of the antimicrobial agent and pharmacokinetic/pharmacodynamic parameters. Drugs such as penicillins and 5-flucytosine have to be dosed more frequently or sometimes as continuous infusion since they exert maximum antibiotic effect when concentration persists above MIC for longer durations. Antibiotics that have long half-lives, such as ceftriaxone allow infrequent dosing to maintain concentrations above MIC for prolonged time. This **time-dependent killing** is also shown by glycopeptides and macrolides [39–41].

Antibiotics such as aminoglycosides, fluoroquinolones, rifampicin show **concentration-dependent killing** and the peak concentration that is reached is most predictive of efficacy. These antibiotics can be administered more intermittently such as once a day at higher dose, despite short half-life. They have a long post-antibiotic effect and effectiveness persists long after antibiotic concentrations fall below the MIC.

For the third group of antibiotics such as Daptomycin, the cumulative dose is most important and daily dosing has no additional effect on efficacy. These antibiotics also have a prolonged PAE.

1.6 Adverse Effects of Antimicrobial Use

> "sola dosis facit venemum"
> —Paracelsus

'cptly applied to the toxicity seen with use of antibiotics. In some cases, drugs which are lifesaving can end up endangering lives. Even at therapeutic doses, antibiotics can cause a variety of adverse effects. A delicate and reasonable balance must be maintained to achieve the best risk to benefit ratio. Various adverse effects resulting from antimicrobial use are depicted in the Fig. 1.2.

1.6.1 Systemic Adverse Effects

Antimicrobial agents can cause dose-dependent organ toxicities. Commonly involved organs are kidney and liver [42, 43]. Major organ toxicities with examples of causative antimicrobials are included in Table 1.6.

1.6.2 Hypersensitivity Reactions

These are unpredictable dose independent reactions which can be caused by any antimicrobial agent. Hypersensitivity reactions are most commonly caused by beta lactam antibiotics and sulfonamides but can also result from macrolides, tetracyclines, fluoroquinolones or any other antimicrobial agent. These reactions can be categorized as immediate or delayed hypersensitivity reactions. Immediate hypersensitivity reactions occur within one hour of administration of antimicrobial agents

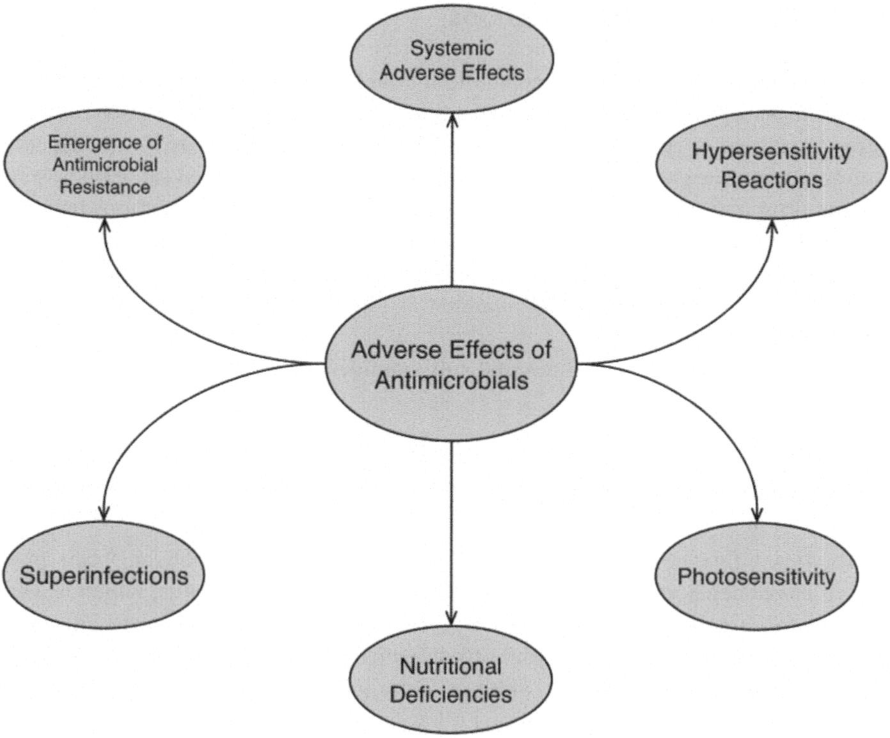

Fig. 1.2 Various adverse effects resulting from antimicrobial use

Table 1.6 Common organ toxicities due to antimicrobials

Organs/system involved	Causal antimicrobial agent
Kidney	Tetracycline, aminoglycoside, vancomycin, polymyxin B, amphotericin B
Haematological/bone marrow	Chloramphenicol, amphotericin B, linezolid, sulfonamides, nitrofurantoin, vancomycin, rifampicin
Ear/vestibulocochlear nerve	Vancomycin, aminoglycoside, erythromycin, chloroquine
Liver	Tetracycline, azithromycin, pyrazinamide, isoniazid, rifampicin
Neurological	Polymyxin B, amphotericin B, ciprofloxacin, imipenem, vancomycin

and are mediated by IgE antibodies. They may be manifested as urticaria, rhinitis, angioedema, bronchospasm or even anaphylactic shock. Delayed hypersensitivity reactions are cell mediated cutaneous reactions that manifest as benign exanthems or severe cutaneous reactions such as drug reaction with eosinophilia and systemic symptoms syndrome, toxic epidermal necrolysis or Stevens Johnson syndrome [44–46].

1.6.3 Photosensitivity Reactions

The interaction of medications and sunlight could lead to photosensitive responses in certain susceptible patients. Photosensitivity reactions can be categorized as phototoxic reactions or photoallergic reactions. Phototoxic reactions are immediate and eruptions occur on exposed skin areas. They are dependent on the dose of photosensitizing drug and intensity of exposure to sunlight. Photoallergic reactions have an immunological basis and require previous exposure to the photosensitizer. These could be immediate (antigen antibody mediated) or delayed (cell mediated) hypersensitivity responses. They could manifest as papulovesicular eruptions, pruritus, and eczematous dermatitis.

Fluoroquinolones, tetracyclines and sulfonamides are the most photoactive antimicrobials [32, 47, 48] (Table 1.7).

1.6.4 Nutritional Deficiencies

Antibiotics influence gut flora activities and xenobiotic metabolism. Their prolonged usage negatively impacts the gut health and nutritional status, which is why they are frequently supplemented with probiotics. They also alter gastrointestinal motility and colon processes, leading to defective absorption. Vitamin K and vitamin B as well as several minerals are most commonly depleted, leading to bleeding diathesis, gastritis and anaemia, among other nutritional problems.

1.6.4.1 Superinfections

Superinfections are second infections that occur in patients taking an antibiotic due to disturbance in the normal microbiome. These are unrelated to the original infection for which the antibiotic was taken. Reduction in the normal microbiome provides an opportunity for a person's own microbiome or pathogenic microbes from the outside environment to grow and cause a new infection. Broad-spectrum antibiotics are more likely to cause superinfections than narrow-spectrum antibiotics. Long duration of antibiotic therapy, poor nutritional status, old age and immunosuppression (caused by corticosteroids, HIV, malignancies etc.) increase the risk of superinfections.

Table 1.7 Common antimicrobials that act as photosensitizers and their type of photosensitivity reaction

Antimicrobials	Photosensitivity reactions
Demeclocycline>chlortetracycline >minocycline>doxycycline	Phototoxic reactions
Lomefloxacin>norfloxacin>ofloxacin	Phototoxic, photoallergic, photomutagenic reactions
Sulfamethoxazole	Phototoxic and photoallergic

- *Clostridium difficile* can occur following treatment with broad spectrum antibiotics such as extended-spectrum cephalosporins and fluoroquinolones. It can cause severe life-threatening diarrhea that can be resistant to commonly used antimicrobials.
- Vaginal or oral thrush is a common superinfection caused by Candida. Candida can often be a part of normal commensal flora but antibiotic treatment disturbs the microbiota balance and causes an increase in their numbers. Fungi can also rarely spread to the blood and cause severe infections.
- An increase in urinary tract infection has also been linked with antibiotic use. Particularly women treated with antibiotics have been found to be five times more likely to acquire a urinary tract infection.
- Preliminary studies have linked antibiotic use to certain severe disease conditions such as obesity by affecting the human microbiome.

1.6.5 Emergence of Antimicrobial Resistance

Antimicrobial resistance means the bacteria can thrive despite the presence of antibiotics at concentrations that normally inhibit or kill the bacteria during standard therapy. Evolution of resistance is inevitable during antimicrobial therapy as the resistant forms are selected.

Misuse and overuse further aggravate the problem of resistance.

Microorganisms can be intrinsically resistant to one or more antibiotics due to evolutionary mechanisms that allow them to naturally thrive with antimicrobial producing organisms in the environment. In clinical settings, this intrinsic resistance does not pose much problem rather acquired resistance where originally susceptible bacteria become resistant is the main concern. The acquired resistance could result from horizontal gene acquisition of foreign genetic determinants of resistance or mutations in chromosomal genes [49–51].

1.6.5.1 Resistance Due to Mutation

A subset of bacteria amongst the susceptible bacteria may develop a mutation that allows them to thrive in the presence of antimicrobial agents. The susceptible bacteria is eliminated while this mutant bacteria is selected and predominates. Mutations may lead to antimicrobial resistance by decreasing the affinity of the antimicrobial drug to the target, decreasing the uptake of the antimicrobial drug, increasing the efflux of antimicrobial drug or causing modifications in the vital metabolic pathways [52].

1.6.5.2 Resistance Due to Gene Transfer

Bacteria may acquire genetic determinants of resistance from other bacteria in the environment. This exchange of genetic material is implicated in the development and spread of resistance to frequently used antimicrobials. The genetic transfer can occur through either of the three processes viz. transformation, transduction or conjugation. In the hospital settings conjugation i.e. cell-to-cell transfer of mobile

Table 1.8 Mechanisms of antimicrobial resistance

<table>
<tr><th colspan="3">Mechanism of resistance</th><th>Examples</th></tr>
<tr><td rowspan="2">Modification of the antibiotic</td><td colspan="2">Enzymatic alteration</td><td>Adenylation, acetylation and phosphorylation of aminoglycosides, acetylation of chloramphenicol, acetylation of streptogramins, adenylation of lincosamides</td></tr>
<tr><td colspan="2">Destruction</td><td>Penicillins by β lactamases</td></tr>
<tr><td rowspan="2">Inability to reach the target</td><td colspan="2">Decreased influx</td><td>β-Lactams, vancomycin, tetracyclines</td></tr>
<tr><td colspan="2">Increased efflux</td><td>Tetracyclines, macrolides, fluoroquinolones, carbapenems, β-lactams, and polymyxins</td></tr>
<tr><td rowspan="4">Altered target</td><td colspan="2">Target protection</td><td>Tetracycline, fluoroquinolones</td></tr>
<tr><td rowspan="2">Target modification</td><td>Mutation</td><td>Rifampicin, fluoroquinolone, oxazolidinone</td></tr>
<tr><td>Enzymatic alteration</td><td>Macrolide (ribosomal methylation), linezolid (Cfr mediated)</td></tr>
<tr><td colspan="2">Target replacement/ bypass</td><td>Methicillin (PBP2a) and vancomycin, cotrimoxazole</td></tr>
<tr><td colspan="3">Cell adaptive mechanisms</td><td>Daptomycin, vancomycin</td></tr>
</table>

genetic elements such as plasmids or transposons is the most prevalent mechanism. Horizontal gene transfer through transposition involves incorporation of naked DNA while transduction is phage mediated.

The various mechanisms by which microorganisms develop resistance to the antimicrobial agents have been summarized in Table 1.8. Further details of antimicrobial resistance have been included in chap. 2.

References

1. UN, global health agencies sound alarm on drug-resistant infections; new recommendations to reduce 'staggering number' of future deaths | UN News [Internet]. [cited 2025 Aug 20]. Available from: https://news.un.org/en/story/2019/04/1037471
2. Pancu DF, Scurtu A, Macasoi IG, Marti D, Mioc M, Soica C, et al. Antibiotics: conventional therapy and natural compounds with antibacterial activity-a pharmaco-toxicological screening. Antibiotics [Internet]. 2021 Apr 1 [cited 2025 Aug 20];10(4). Available from: https://pubmed.ncbi.nlm.nih.gov/33917092/
3. Krause KM, Serio AW, Kane TR, Connolly LE. Aminoglycosides: An overview. Cold Spring Harb Perspect Med [Internet]. 2016 Jun 1 [cited 2025 Aug 20];6(6). Available from: https://pubmed.ncbi.nlm.nih.gov/27252397/
4. Kim D, Kim S, Kwon Y, Kim Y, Park H, Kwak K, et al. Structural Insights for β-Lactam Antibiotics. Biomol Ther (Seoul) [Internet]. 2023 [cited 2025 Aug 20];31(2):141–147. Available from: https://pubmed.ncbi.nlm.nih.gov/36788654/
5. Cephalosporins—PubMed [Internet]. [cited 2025 Aug 20]. Available from: https://pubmed.ncbi.nlm.nih.gov/31855361/
6. Trimethoprim | C14H18N4O3 | CID 5578—PubChem [Internet]. [cited 2025 Aug 20]. Available from: https://pubchem.ncbi.nlm.nih.gov/compound/Trimethoprim
7. Kang HK, Park Y. Glycopeptide antibiotics: structure and mechanisms of action. J Bacteriol Virol [Internet] 2015 Jun 1 [cited 2025 Aug 20];45(2):67–78. Available from: https://synapse.koreamed.org/articles/1034205

8. Jednačak T, Mikulandra I, Novak P. Advanced methods for studying structure and interactions of macrolide antibiotics. Int J Mol Sci [Internet] 2020 Oct 2 [cited 2025 Aug 20];21(20):1–27. Available from: https://pubmed.ncbi.nlm.nih.gov/33096889/
9. Metronidazole | C6H9N3O3 | CID 4173—PubChem [Internet]. [cited 2025 Aug 20]. Available from: https://pubchem.ncbi.nlm.nih.gov/compound/Metronidazole
10. Linezolid | C16H20FN3O4 | CID 441401—PubChem [Internet]. [cited 2025 Aug 20]. Available from: https://pubchem.ncbi.nlm.nih.gov/compound/Linezolid
11. Chloramphenicol | C11H12Cl2N2O5 | CID 5959—PubChem [Internet]. [cited 2025 Aug 20]. Available from: https://pubchem.ncbi.nlm.nih.gov/compound/Chloramphenicol
12. Correia S, Poeta P, Hébraud M, Capelo JL, Igrejas G. Mechanisms of quinolone action and resistance: where do we stand? J Med Microbiol [Internet] 2017 May 1 [cited 2025 Aug 20];66(5):551–559. Available from: https://pubmed.ncbi.nlm.nih.gov/28504927/
13. Kocsis B, Domokos J, Szabo D. Chemical structure and pharmacokinetics of novel quinolone agents represented by avarofloxacin, delafloxacin, finafloxacin, zabofloxacin and nemonoxacin. Ann Clin Microbiol Antimicrob [Internet]. 2016 May 23 [cited 2025 Aug 20];15(1). Available from: https://pubmed.ncbi.nlm.nih.gov/27215369/
14. Ghani S, Khan N, Sable H, Yao F, Shafiq M. Computational techniques for enhancing PK/PD modeling and simulation and ADMET prediction. Computational Methods in Medicinal Chemistry, Pharmacology, and Toxicology [Internet]. 2025 Jan 1 [cited 2025 Aug 9];153–174. Available from: https://linkinghub.elsevier.com/retrieve/pii/B9780443330247000011
15. Lamb HM, Figgitt DP, Faulds D. Quinupristin/dalfopristin: a review of its use in the management of serious gram-positive infections. Drugs [Internet] 1999 [cited 2025 Aug 20];58(6):1061–1097. Available from: https://pubmed.ncbi.nlm.nih.gov/10651391/
16. Mast Y, Wohlleben W. Streptogramins—two are better than one! Int J Med Microbiol [Internet] 2014 Jan [cited 2025 Aug 20];304(1):44–50. Available from: https://pubmed.ncbi.nlm.nih.gov/24119565/
17. Ovung A, Bhattacharyya J. Sulfonamide drugs: structure, antibacterial property, toxicity, and biophysical interactions. Biophys Rev [Internet] 2021 Apr 1 [cited 2025 Aug 20];13(2):259. Available from: https://pmc.ncbi.nlm.nih.gov/articles/PMC8046889/
18. Kelly TE, Hackett PH. Acetazolamide and sulfonamide allergy: a not so simple story. High Alt Med Biol [Internet] 2010 Dec 1 [cited 2025 Aug 20];11(4):319–323. Available from: https://pubmed.ncbi.nlm.nih.gov/21190500/
19. Chopra I, Roberts M. Tetracycline antibiotics: mode of action, applications, molecular biology, and epidemiology of bacterial resistance. Microbiol Mol Biol Rev [Internet] 2001 Jun [cited 2025 Aug 20];65(2):232–260. Available from: https://pubmed.ncbi.nlm.nih.gov/11381101/
20. Tacconelli E, Carrara E, Savoldi A, Harbarth S, Mendelson M, Monnet DL et al (2018) Discovery, research, and development of new antibiotics: the WHO priority list of antibiotic-resistant bacteria and tuberculosis. Lancet Infect Dis 18(3):318–327
21. Vasilie S, Manea F, Baciu A, Pop A (2018) Dual use of boron-doped diamond electrode in antibiotics-containing water treatment and process control. Process Saf Environ Prot 117:446–453
22. Chaudhary V, Rustagi S, Kaushik A, Bhutani M. Perspective—Prospect of Nano-enabled optical biosensors for antibiotic abuse surveillance as an early prevention tool for antimicrobial resistance. ECS J Solid State Sci Technol [Internet] 2024 Jan 17 [cited 2025 Aug 18];13(1):017003. Available from: https://iopscience.iop.org/article/10.1149/2162-8777/ad1c8d
23. Chaudhary V, Rustagi S, … AKEJ of S, 2024 undefined. Perspective—Prospect of Nano-Enabled Optical Biosensors for Antibiotic Abuse Surveillance as an Early Prevention Tool for Antimicrobial Resistance. iopscience.iop.org [Internet]. [cited 2025 Jan 7]; Available from: https://iopscience.iop.org/article/10.1149/2162-8777/ad1c8d/meta
24. Chaudhary N, Verma D, Yadav AK, Sharma JG, Solanki PR (2023) Rational hydrothermal-assisted green synthesis of blueish emitting carbon dots as an optical sensing platform for antibiotic detection in the milk sample. Talanta Open 8:100259

25. Wang S, Li C, Yin H, Gao B, Yu Z, Zhou Y et al (2025) A novel Ag/Bi/Bi2O2CO3 photocatalyst effectively removes antibiotic-resistant bacteria and tetracycline from water under visible light irradiation. Environ Res 264:120313
26. Roose-Amsaleg C, Laverman AM. Do antibiotics have environmental side-effects? Impact of synthetic antibiotics on biogeochemical processes. Environmental Science and Pollution Research [Internet] 2016 Mar 1 [cited 2025 Jul 30];23(5):4000–4012. Available from: https://link.springer.com/article/10.1007/s11356-015-4943-3
27. Andersson DI, Hughes D (2014) Microbiological effects of sublethal levels of antibiotics. Nat Rev Microbiol 12(7):465–478
28. Chaudhary V, Khanna V, Ahmed Awan HT, Singh K, Khalid M, Mishra YK, et al. Towards hospital-on-chip supported by 2D MXenes-based 5th generation intelligent biosensors. Biosens Bioelectron [Internet]. 2023 Jan 15 [cited 2025 Jun 4];220:114847. Available from: https://www.sciencedirect.com/science/article/pii/S0956566322008879
29. Bhadola P, Chaudhary V, Markandan K, Talreja RK, Aggarwal S, Nigam K, et al. Analysing role of airborne particulate matter in abetting SARS-CoV-2 outbreak for scheming regional pandemic regulatory modalities. Environ Res [Internet]. 2023 Nov 1 [cited 2025 Jun 7];236:116646. Available from: https://www.sciencedirect.com/science/article/abs/pii/S0013935123014500?via%3Dihub
30. Talreja RK, Sable H, Chaudhary V, Kadian S, Singh Mamta, Kishore J, et al. Challenges in lab-to-clinic translation of 5th/6th generation intelligent nanomaterial-enabled biosensors. ECS Sensors Plus [Internet] 2024 Dec 16 [cited 2024 Dec 21]; Available from: https://iopscience.iop.org/article/10.1149/2754-2726/ad9f7e
31. Singh V, Kasana E, Batra J, Sable H, Saxena R. Antimicrobial Resistance: Mechanisms, Screening Techniques and Biosensors. J Pharm Negat Results [Internet]. 2022 Oct 12 [cited 2025 Aug 18];13:1724–1735. Available from: https://pnrjournal.com/index.php/home/article/view/2049
32. Ramezani Farani M, Farsadrooh M, Zare I, Gholami A, Akhavan O. Green Synthesis of Magnesium Oxide Nanoparticles and Nanocomposites for Photocatalytic Antimicrobial, Antibiofilm and Antifungal Applications. Catalysts 2023, Vol 13, Page 642 [Internet]. 2023 Mar 23 [cited 2024 May 25];13(4):642. Available from: https://www.mdpi.com/2073-4344/13/4/642/htm
33. Devadas S, Zakaria Z, Shariff M, Bhassu S, Aquaculture MK, 2023 undefined. Methodologies and standards for monitoring antimicrobial use and antimicrobial resistance in shrimp aquaculture. Elsevier [Internet]. [cited 2025 Jan 7]; Available from: https://www.sciencedirect.com/science/article/pii/S0044848623009900
34. Ramzan M, Raza A, … Z un NTT in, 2024 undefined. Detection of antimicrobial resistance (AMR) and antimicrobial susceptibility testing (AST) using advanced spectroscopic techniques: A review. Elsevier [Internet]. [cited 2025 Jan 7]; Available from: https://www.sciencedirect.com/science/article/pii/S016599362400044X
35. Kaprou GD, Bergšpica I, Alexa EA, Alvarez-Ordóñez A, Prieto M. Rapid methods for antimicrobial resistance diagnostics. mdpi.com [Internet]. 2021 [cited 2025 Jan 7]; Available from: https://www.mdpi.com/2079-6382/10/2/209
36. Aarestrup FM, Woolhouse MEJ. Using sewage for surveillance of antimicrobial resistance. Science (1979). 2020 Feb 7;367(6478):630–632
37. Rawson TM, Wilson RC, O'Hare D, Herrero P, Kambugu A, Lamorde M, et al. Optimizing antimicrobial use: challenges, advances and opportunities. Nat Rev Microbiol 2021 19:12 [Internet]. 2021 Jun 22 [cited 2025 Jan 8];19(12):747–758. Available from: https://www.nature.com/articles/s41579-021-00578-9
38. Durazzi F, Pezzani MD, Arieti F, Simonetti O, Canziani LM, Carrara E, et al. Modelling antimicrobial resistance transmission to guide personalized antimicrobial stewardship interventions and infection control policies in healthcare setting: a pilot study. Scientific Reports 2023 13:1 [Internet]. 2023 Sep 22 [cited 2025 Jan 7];13(1):1–10. Available from: https://www.nature.com/articles/s41598-023-42511-5

39. Sable H, Vaishali, Singh V. β2-microglobulin biomarkers' roles in assessing cadmium toxicity. Int J Med Toxicol Legal Med. 2023 Jul 1;26(3 and 4):112–116
40. Michael CA, Dominey-Howes D, Labbate M. The antimicrobial resistance crisis: causes, consequences, and management. Front Public Health 2014 Sep 16;2(SEP)
41. Christaki E, Marcou M, Tofarides A (2020) Antimicrobial resistance in bacteria: mechanisms, evolution, and persistence. J Mol Evol 88(1):26–40
42. Sable H, Singh V, Kumar V, Roy A, Pandit S, Kaur K, et al. Toxicological and bioremediation profiling of nonessential heavy metals (mercury, chromium, cadmium, aluminium) and their impact on human health: A review. Toxicologie Analytique et Clinique [Internet]. 2024; Available from: https://linkinghub.elsevier.com/retrieve/pii/S2352007824001185
43. Adator EH, Narvaez-Bravo C, Zaheer R, Cook SR, Tymensen L, Hannon SJ et al (2020) A one health comparative assessment of antimicrobial resistance in generic and extended-spectrum cephalosporin-resistant escherichia coli from beef production, sewage and clinical settings. Microorganisms 8(6):1–22
44. Shortridge D, Streit JM, Mendes R, Castanheira M (2022) In Vitro Activity of Cefiderocol against U.S. and European Gram-Negative Clinical Isolates Collected in 2020 as Part of the SENTRY Antimicrobial Surveillance Program. Microbiol Spectr. 10(2)
45. Mohamed A, Atta RR, Kotp AA, Abo El-Ela FI, Abd El-Raheem H, Farghali A, et al. Green synthesis and characterization of iron oxide nanoparticles for the removal of heavy metals (Cd2+ and Ni2+) from aqueous solutions with Antimicrobial Investigation. Scientific Reports 2023 13:1 [Internet]. 2023 May 4 [cited 2024 Jun 23];13(1):1–30. Available from: https://www.nature.com/articles/s41598-023-31704-7
46. Kanimozhi S, Hariram M, Ganesan V, Muthuramkumar S, Vivekanandhan S. Exploring Azadirachta indica Gum as the Sustainable Fuel in Combustion Process for the Synthesis of ZnO Nanoparticles with Antimicrobial and Antioxidant Potentials. https://doi.org/101142/S1793984423500046 [Internet]. 2023 Mar 15 [cited 2024 May 29];13(2). Available from: https://www.worldscientific.com/worldscinet/nl
47. Rani N, Yadav S, Mushtaq A, Rani S, Saini M, Rawat S, et al. Azadirachta indica peel extract-mediated synthesis of ZnO nanoparticles for antimicrobial, supercapacitor and photocatalytic applications. Chemical Papers [Internet]. 2024 Apr 1 [cited 2024 May 29];78(6):3687–3704. Available from: https://link.springer.com/article/10.1007/s11696-024-03340-6
48. Aram Z, Divya, Yadav K, Ashu, Yadav S, Sable H, et al. Azadirachta Indica-Assisted Sustainable Green ZnO Nanoparticles for Diversified Applications. 2025 [cited 2025 Aug 18];227–251. Available from: https://link.springer.com/chapter/10.1007/978-981-96-5166-5_16
49. Murray CJ, Ikuta KS, Sharara F, Swetschinski L, Robles Aguilar G, Gray A, et al. Global burden of bacterial antimicrobial resistance in 2019: a systematic analysis. Lancet 2022 Feb 12;399(10325):629–655
50. Rabiee N, Ahmadi S, Akhavan O, Luque R (2022) Silver and gold nanoparticles for antimicrobial purposes against multi-drug resistance bacteria. Materials 15(5)
51. Sable H, Kumar V, Mishra R, Kumar S, pandit S, Singh V, et al. Biosorption of hexavalent chromium by Shewanella putrefaciens MTCC 8104: response surface methodology optimization and mechanistic insights. Indian J Microbiol [Internet] 2024 Aug 9 [cited 2024 Sep 28];1–17. Available from: https://link.springer.com/article/10.1007/s12088-024-01365-9
52. Rani A, Kaur G, Kumar R, Sachan RSK, Kumar M, Sable H, et al. Role of DNA Methylation in the Pathogenesis of Skin Disorders: Mechanisms, Inhibitors of Methylation-Related Enzyme, and Molecular Docking Studies. Biomed Res Int [Internet]. 2025 Jan 1 [cited 2025 Jul 23];2025(1):7002918. Available from: https://doi.org/10.1155/bmri/7002918

Antibiotic Abuse as a Precursor to Antimicrobial Resistance

2

Rahul Kumar, Pankaj Gautam, Navin Kumar, Tanja Vasić, and Debasis Mitra

2.1 Introduction

Antibiotics, also known as antimicrobials, are used to treat diseases in both humans and animals by either killing or inhibiting the growth of disease-causing microorganisms [1]. Antimicrobials, which include antibiotics, antifungals, antivirals, anthelmintics, and more, are essential for the health and welfare of both people and animals. The discovery of antibiotics has been one of the most significant and influential medical achievements. The antibiotic era started more than a century ago with the discovery of the first known antibiotic, Salvarsan, in 1910. In 1928, Alexander Fleming, a bacteriology professor at London's St. Mary's Hospital, accidentally discovered penicillin by separating it from mold juice. Fleming first thought that penicillin might be used as a local antiseptic, notwithstanding its inability to purify it or pinpoint its characteristics of action. Flemings of penicillin publications, however, provided the foundation for more antimicrobial research at the University of Oxford in 1939, leading to the discovery of other antibiotic classes and the identification of next-generation penicillins. Similar to the worldwide effort to develop vaccines against the COVID-19 pandemic, it was first used in the final year of World War II and led to a global push to commercially manufacture pure penicillins. Owing to its strong bacteriostatic properties, chloramphenicol was developed in the 1940s and has excellent therapeutic benefits. Two third-generation aminopenicillins

R. Kumar · P. Gautam · D. Mitra (✉)
Department of Microbiology, Graphic Era (Deemed to be University), Dehradun, Uttarakhand, India

N. Kumar
Department of Biotechnology, Graphic Era (Deemed to be University), Dehradun, Uttarakhand, India

T. Vasić
Faculty of Agriculture, University of Niš, Kruševac, Serbia

V. Chaudhary, N. Bhalla (eds.), *Biosensors for Tackling Antimicrobial Resistance (AMR)*, https://doi.org/10.1007/978-981-95-9151-0_2

that are still used today are ampicillin and amoxicillin, which were first introduced in the 1960s. AMR, or antimicrobial resistance, was discovered in the 1940s shortly after the discovery of penicillin. Specific *E. coli* strains may be capable of producing penicillinase, thereby nullifying the therapeutic action of the antibiotic. Thereafter, some *S. aureus* and *S. pneumoniae* strains were found to be resistant to the drug. Methicillin-resistant *S. aureus* is often called a "SUPERBUG" because it produces numerous virulence factors. MRSA may evolve into new strains with increased virulence and colonization ability to maximize gene content and expression [2, 3]. The supply of antibiotics has reversed from the initial patterns as the demand remains high because of the prevalence of antibiotics in the current market. The number of people who receive antibiotics is now high owing to their overuse, since they are often not really needed. Unfortunately, this has led to the emergence of AMR, which has gradually eroded the potency of these drugs. Bacteria can become resistant to antibiotics each time they are used. According to the World Health Organization, antibiotics have already reached the end of their useful lives, and if nothing is done, we will soon enter a post-antibiotic era in which common illnesses and minor wounds can become deadly once more. If treatment is not received, antimicrobial resistance (AMR) can surpass diabetes and cancer as the world's most pressing health issues, posing an enormous threat to global public health. Antibiotic abuse and the implications of the rise in antibiotic prescriptions for viral infections such as influenza or the common cold, which antibiotics cannot treat and instead contribute to the proliferation of resistant bacteria, is one aspect of AMR that impacts human health. As soon as they started feeling better, patients stopped taking antibiotics before completing the prescribed course, leaving behind germs that could develop resistance and lead to more difficult-to-cure recurrent illnesses. Broad-spectrum antibiotics kill both beneficial and pathogenic bacteria. This results in microbial imbalance, causing resistance and secondary infections, such as *Clostridium difficile*, where a narrow-spectrum antibiotic would have been sufficient. Other ways in which antibiotics are misused include obtaining drugs illegally or using leftover prescription drugs because the drug is not appropriate for the condition. This results in resistance. In agriculture, antibiotics are commonly used to enhance the growth and maintain healthy livestock healthy. Humans may contract resistant bacteria through the environment, direct contact, or the food chain. Resistant infections by MRSA or carbapenem-resistant *Enterobacteriaceae* (CRE) pose major challenges within hospitals and other healthcare sectors and frequently lead to severe cases of illness and death since there might not be appropriate treatments that can be offered to infected patients [4–6]. The above scenarios illustrate how improper use of antibiotics in human and agricultural medicine affects the efficacy of treatment and health status and becomes part of the growing threat of antimicrobial resistance.

2.2 Mechanisms of Antimicrobial Resistance

The source of antimicrobial resistance, a threat to global health, is microorganisms adapted to survive exposure to antimicrobial medications. This may occur naturally over time due to genetic mutations or the acquisition of resistance genes; however, human activity, specifically the abuse and overuse of antibiotics, has dramatically accelerated this process. AMR can be acquired by horizontal gene transfer, genetic alterations, or the intrinsic natural characteristics of some microbes. Because of AMR, traditional therapies are less effective, which increases the risk of complications, hospital stays, and deaths, prolongs infections, and limits treatment alternatives. Methicillin-resistant *Staphylococcus aureus* (MRSA) and carbapenem-resistant *Enterobacteriaceae* (CRE) are two examples of multidrug-resistant organisms (MDROs) that it helps spread. There are various uses for genetic and phenotypic resistance to microorganisms. Microorganisms use mechanisms that do not come under the effect of some drugs, endure selective pressure, and multiply. In a word, the genetic resistance can be summarized into the following strategies: horizontal gene transfer, alteration, enzymatic degradation or chemical modification, efflux pump, decreased permeability, biofilm development, dormancy and persistence, mutation within the DNA of the microorganism. Inappropriate broad-spectrum antibiotic use, incomplete courses, self-medication, excessive use in agriculture, environmental contamination, overprescription in healthcare, and the use of inferior or fake medicines are factors in the emergence and spread of AMR. Antibiotics are prematurely stopped in incomplete courses, leaving partially treated infections untreated, and fostering the growth of resistant microorganisms. Self-medication, frequently with improper dosages or durations, worsens the development of drug resistance. Other factors that cause AMR include overuse in agriculture, hospitals, and pharmaceutical factory waste and the use of low-quality or counterfeit antibiotics [7–9]. Therefore, it is important to understand how resistance occurs to fight AMR and preserve the effectiveness of antimicrobials. We can attempt to limit the spread of AMR and ensure the security and effectiveness of antibiotics for future generations by understanding their resistance mechanisms (Fig. 2.1).

2.3 Impacts of Antibiotic Abuse on Public Health

The overuse and misuse of antibiotics, popularly referred to as antibiotic abuse, have adverse effects on public health. These include increased resistance to disease, higher medical expenses, and financial distress. The abuse of antibiotics directly leads to the growth of multidrug-resistant organisms (MDROs). This leads to increased morbidity and mortality. Common MDROs include MDR-TB, Mycobacterium tuberculosis, CRE, VRE, and MRSA. Treatment of resistant infections is cumbersome and often requires long-term treatment. More than 1.2 million fatalities are directly attributed to the burden of AMR, while indirectly, over five million deaths are accounted for worldwide. The prevalence of resistant infections

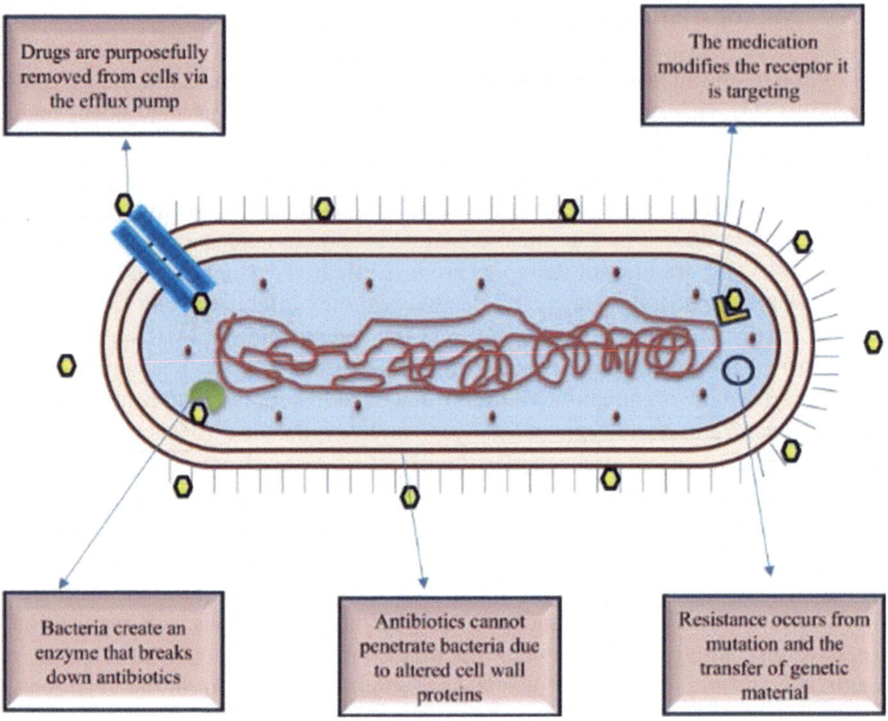

Fig. 2.1 Mechanisms of resistance

increases with uncontrolled accessibility of antibiotics and poor sanitation. AMR and antibiotic misuse incur huge financial costs to individuals, health systems, and global economies. Some direct healthcare costs include expensive second-line or last-resort antibiotics, extended hospital stay, additional diagnostic testing, and critical care. The increased demand for diagnostic equipment, specialist therapies, and infection control measures brought about by resistant illnesses strains in public health budgets. Examples of indirect costs may include higher mortality rates as well as lost output owing to prolonged diseases that, in turn, might impact global GDP, reaching as much as 3.8% by 2050. Because of anxiety over the spread of resistant infections, AMR also affects agriculture and inhibits international travel and trade. Diminishing investment in health structures and economic growth poses issues for countries with significant AMR burdens. The most vulnerable populations, including the elderly, people with weakened immune systems, and those living in LMICs, are most affected by resistant diseases, thereby perpetuating public health disparities. Unequal access to effective treatment exacerbates health disparities [10–13]. AMR threatens global health security by undermining five decades of progress in the treatment of infectious diseases (Table 2.1).

Table 2.1 Antibiotic abuse as a precursor to AMR

Factors	Specifies
Overexpose and hospital use	Hospitals utilize antibiotics a lot especially as a preventive precaution
Inadequate treatment compliance	As their symptoms get better patients quit taking antibiotics but often do not finish the course
The use of fake medications	In low-income areas counterfeit or inferior antibiotics are available
Inadequate regulatory monitoring	Absence of stringent laws controlling the distribution of antibiotics
Take care of oneself	Non prescribed antibiotic use by patients results in insufficient treatment
Abuse in farming	Widespread use of antibiotics in animals to prevent sickness and promote growth
Insufficient patient knowledge	False beliefs regarding the use of antibiotics to treat viral illnesses such as colds
Overprescription drugs use	Prescriptions for antibiotics in the absence of verified bacterial illnesses

2.3.1 Antibiotics in Agriculture and AMR Development

In agriculture, antibiotics are extensively used in animal husbandry, fisheries, cattle, and poultry. They assist in the prevention and treatment of a variety of crop diseases in the agricultural industry, even though their main role in cattle and animal husbandry is typically to promote growth and fight infections. Antimicrobial resistance develops and spreads owing to the use of antibiotics in veterinary medicine. Better control of the use of antibiotics in animals, particularly those that are also used in human medicine, is necessary to maintain their effectiveness. Critical and highly important antibiotics should be used cautiously. CIAs are necessary when first-line antibiotics have not been able to treat a disease. There is a great risk to the treatment and control of diseases globally because it seems unlikely that any new antibiotics will soon be available. In addition to being a global public health issue, it affects the environment, food security, and animal health. Antibiotics need to be accessible and applied so that animal welfare, health, and productivity can be preserved and nutritious and safe food can be produced. If antibiotics become ineffective, farmers will not have the right medication to protect the health and welfare of their animals [14–16]. Farm profitability and productivity are adversely affected. Veterinary drugs such as antimicrobial medicines play a vital role in promoting global public health through animal health and welfare. Animal illnesses contribute to 20% of the output losses. Thus, the preservation of the efficacy of antibiotic medicines cannot be overstated. With the increase in the world's population, there is a higher demand for high-quality animal protein, including eggs, meat, and milk, thus emphasizing the need to preserve the effectiveness of antibiotics. Over the past 20 years, the World Organization for Animal Health (WOAH) has been actively fighting antibiotic resistance using a comprehensive "one health" approach to safeguard the health of people, animals, plants, and the environment. The primary goals of WOAH's strategy are to, among other things, support effective governance and capacity building regarding animal health and welfare, promote careful handling of antimicrobial products, push for the adoption of international standards, and raise public awareness and understanding of antimicrobial resistance through targeted advocacy and communication campaigns [17–20].

2.3.2 Control & Trends

The first step in tackling AMR in agriculture is the establishment of a global target to reduce the use of antibiotics and limit the types of antibiotics used, that is, those used for human health. The use of antibiotics in water or animal feed for purposes other than prevention should be prohibited. The objective should be a worldwide environment in which human and animal health and well-being are preserved through food and agricultural systems that minimize the use of antibiotics and associated drugs. Promote improved husbandry and ban all routine uses of antibiotics in agriculture, including withholding prophylactic mass therapy. This implies that farm animals grow under conditions that give way to their welfare and health. Third, superior production of antimicrobials, including waste disposal techniques, must be in place to eliminate such waste from the environment, which is an issue related to industrial pollution. Stressed animals show an increased rate of disease progression. Stress can stimulate hormones such as cortisol, which impair the immune system and reduce immunity. Rather than being robust and naturally resistant to diseases, animals used in intensive agricultural systems are often bred for production. In addition, it can take years for the development of new antibiotics, so efforts to facilitate their discovery must be made. This problem should be addressed at present, rather than waiting for a major catastrophe to force the development of a new antibiotic [21–24].

One area in which this can occur is to provide more support for productive drug development through centralized public clinical trial platforms. Better information exchange at the early stages of AMR development and harmonization of innovative development standards can also be introduced because they can lower the risk or harm to general safety. It might be possible to more successfully support the discovery of new antibiotics by implementing these simple tactics. COVID19 is also perceived to have increased the worldwide threat of AMR, since most cases and treatment programs in some nations require antibiotics to lower the rate of secondary bacterial or fungal infections that may arise. Another need is to consider vaccination as a possible mechanism for offering immunity against medication resistance. Pandemics and epidemics are fought by vaccines. Further research may reveal that vaccines can combat AMR and decrease infection cases that require antibiotic treatment. The COVID-19 pandemic has raised the importance of strong health systems coupled with collaboration across all domains, including medical, scientific, political, regulatory, and social. Drug resistance and infectious diseases have become more prominent in the public mind because of the pandemic. We believe that the key pillars of the health system in managing antibiotic resistance are prevention and control, monitoring and data creation, awareness and behavioural change through education and campaigns, and access and conservation (including diagnostics, recommendations, and legislation). Every country must work together to take greater responsibility for the use and administration of antibiotics within its borders. With its approach toward health systems and raising proper funding to coordinate different programmatic efforts, the WHO could bolster its leadership in combating AMR (Swenson 2024). The funding for programs to achieve the SDGs, universal health coverage, water, sanitation, and hygiene should consider antimicrobial resistance. Among the 52 normative recommendations prepared in the last 5 years, the most significant contribution comes from the WHO Priority Pathogen List. All these suggestions are made to provide for further research and development on antibiotics while ensuring that added challenges would stimulate attention towards new antibiotics and evaluation so that new antibiotics can integrate easily into health systems while ensuring fair access without repeating similar errors in antibiotic overuse and abuse [25–28].

2.4 Strategies to Combat Antibiotic Abuse

Global health is under severe threat owing to the overuse of antibiotics, and one of the biggest concerns is antimicrobial resistance. This problem requires strong policies, cooperative international initiatives, health-focused programs, and public education to form a complex strategy to solve it. To fight antibiotic misuse, international organizations and coalitions have also contributed greatly to creating approaches that stress policy harmonization, intensified surveillance, and support resource-poor areas. The World Health Organization established the Global Action Plan on Antimicrobial Resistance GAP-AMR in 2015, with five strategic objectives: increased knowledge and awareness of AMR, enhancement of knowledge through research and surveillance, infection rates, lowering infection rates through infection prevention and hygiene, optimization of the use of antimicrobial agents in human and animal health, and sustainable investment in the fight against AMR. The Fleming Fund facilitates the improvement of surveillance systems regarding AMR in LMICs, and the One Health Approach addresses antibiotic usage from human, animal, and environmental perspectives. The Antibiotic Resistance Coalition pushes alternative therapies, reduced antibiotic misuse in agriculture, and access to antibiotics on equitable bases. The European Union sets out strict prescription-only sales, bans the use of antibiotics as growth promoters for cattle, and finances scientific investigation through Horizon Europe programs. Hospitals, outpatient clinics, and long-term care facilities are some of the implementation settings for ASPs that are crucial in optimizing antibiotic use while reducing resistance. ASPs ensure that antibiotics are prescribed appropriately only when necessary and at the right dose and duration. Other important elements of ASPs include multidisciplinary teams, monitoring and feedback, restriction policies, and guideline development. Patient education, advocacy, and ethical prescription practices by healthcare providers play a crucial role in the fight against antibiotic abuse (Table 2.2). Antibiotic abuse can

Table 2.2 Effects of antibiotic abuse on public health

Effects	Information
Risk to the security of food	Livestock with resistant infections are less productive and more susceptible to zoonotic illnesses
Global resistant strain spread	Antimicrobial resistance strains that spread by migration, trade and travel
Decreased efficiency of essential antibiotics	Reduction in the effectiveness of life-saving antibiotics for patients undergoing chemotherapy, surgery, and transplantation
Effect on the microbiota	Disruption in the gut flora which can result in Clostridium difficile and other secondary illnesses
The financial burden	High expenses for healthcare systems because of costly second line treatments and prolonged treatments
Higher death tolls	Infections that cannot be treated increase the risk of death
Extended hospitalization and illness	Longer hospital stays and more medical expenses are associated with patients who have resistant infections
The emergence of superbugs	Creation of strains of bacteria that are resistant to many drugs such as MRSA, CRE, and MDR-TB
An increase in antimicrobial resistance	Increased pathogen resistance which makes treating infections more difficult

be addressed through patient communication, rational prescriptions, and policy change advocacy. However, for physicians, the lack of time for consultations, uncertainty in the diagnosis, and pressure from the patient to prescribe antibiotics needlessly are barriers. Public awareness and education are necessary to reduce the abuse of antibiotics. Campaigns and outreach such as World Antimicrobial Awareness Week (WAAW), community outreach, involvement of media, information available for instruction, school activities can increase awareness for AMR and promote the best practices [29–33]. The greatest difficulties were reaching groups with limited health literacy, dispelling myths, and sustaining interest and engagement over time.

2.5 Future Directions and Challenges in Addressing Antibiotic Abuse

This global issue demands innovative solutions, strict legislation, and international cooperation. This demands a multi-faceted approach, as antibiotic resistance evolves and new usage patterns emerge. Rising antibiotic resistance is a critical problem because MDROs multiply across the globe. Overuse of last-resort antibiotics, especially in countries with lax oversight, exacerbates this trend (Limato 2023). Humans can develop resistance against zoonotic bacteria in animals. In most low- and middle-income countries, unregulated access to antibiotics promotes misuse and allows antibiotic resistance genes to be shared across microbial communities throughout the world. The development of antibiotic resistance is further enhanced by non-conventional sources of antibiotics such as counterfeit drugs. Antibiotic resistance genes are stored in reservoirs across natural ecosystems due to environmental pollution from the production of pharmaceuticals, farming, and hospital waste.

Antibiotics are often wrongly prescribed for secondary infections due to ambiguous diagnostics during major health emergencies, such as COVID-19. Resistance patterns display a geospatial approach that has been changing within LMICs, although previously uncommon resistant strains suddenly increased because of laxity in regulation and high use. Expanded use because of the middle class encourages self-medication and careless use in LMICs. Agriculture and veterinary care trends are also increasing. In Asia, antibiotic use in aquaculture has rapidly increased. There is a grave risk to both the environment and public health when antibiotic-resistant bacteria are present in agricultural runoff. Some of the regulatory gaps in combating antibiotic abuse include limited research and innovation, social and economic barriers, limits in diagnosis, and behavioural and cultural variables. Worldwide and globally, organizations that include the World Health Organization focus on bettering frameworks in relation to regulatory control of the use and trading of antibiotics, promoting stewardship of antimicrobials, researching and developing, raising awareness in society, regulating the usage of antibiotics in agriculture, developing innovative diagnostics, and strengthening environmental control.

2.6 Conclusion

This danger, if not arrested and curbed, is significant and has a powerful influence on the entire earth. Disregarding this developing and present global threat is the only factor that can create more problems. Overuse or inappropriate use of antibiotics in agriculture must be lessened to alleviate and combat the growing challenge against the increasing threat of antibiotic resistance as well as the onset of AMR. Evidence for this is found in the well-established lack of regulation over the supply of antibiotics to the agricultural industry and their use in human medicine. While some nations have atoned, more needs to be done to improve animal care and husbandry to lower the incidence of diseases and the demand for antibiotics. Therefore, the world may enforce policies that can be applied to end AMR if the global community continues to work together to address this problem. More than anything, scientific and governing bodies of the world need to work together to establish and implement practical plans. Thus, this may be a way to combat this emerging threat.

References

1. Aram Z, Divya, Yadav K, Ashu, Yadav S, Sable H et al (2025) Azadirachta Indica-assisted sustainable green ZnO nanoparticles for diversified applications. [cited 2025 Aug 18];227–251. Available from: https://link.springer.com/chapter/10.1007/978-981-96-5166-5_16
2. Adator EH, Narvaez-Bravo C, Zaheer R, Cook SR, Tymensen L, Hannon SJ et al (2020) A one health comparative assessment of antimicrobial resistance in generic and extended-spectrum cephalosporin-resistant escherichia coli from beef production, sewage and clinical settings. Microorganisms 8(6):1–22

3. Sable H, Kumar V, Mishra R, Kumar S, Pandit S, Singh V et al (2024) Biosorption of hexavalent chromium by Shewanella putrefaciens MTCC 8104: response surface methodology optimization and mechanistic insights. Indian J Microbiol [Internet] [cited 2025 Aug 19];1–17. Available from: https://link.springer.com/article/10.1007/s12088-024-01365-9
4. Ramezani Farani M, Farsadrooh M, Zare I, Gholami A, Akhavan O (2023) Green synthesis of magnesium oxide nanoparticles and nanocomposites for photocatalytic antimicrobial, antibiofilm and antifungal applications. Catalysts [Internet] [cited 2024 May 25];13(4):642. Available from: https://www.mdpi.com/2073-4344/13/4/642/htm
5. Nejati M, Rostami M, Mirzaei H, Rahimi-Nasrabadi M, Vosoughifar M, Nasab AS et al (2022) Green methods for the preparation of MgO nanomaterials and their drug delivery, anti-cancer and anti-bacterial potentials: a review. Inorg Chem Commun 136:109107
6. Tacconelli E, Carrara E, Savoldi A, Harbarth S, Mendelson M, Monnet DL et al (2018) Discovery, research, and development of new antibiotics: the WHO priority list of antibiotic-resistant bacteria and tuberculosis. Lancet Infect Dis 18(3):318–327
7. Pathania D, Kumar S, Thakur P, Chaudhary V, Kaushik A, Varma RS et al (2022) Essential oil-mediated biocompatible magnesium nanoparticles with enhanced antibacterial, antifungal, and photocatalytic efficacies. Sci Rep [Internet] [cited 2024 May 25];12(1):1–13. Available from: https://www.nature.com/articles/s41598-022-14984-3
8. Chaudhary V, Rustagi S, Kaushik A, Bhutani M (2024) Perspective—prospect of nano-enabled optical biosensors for antibiotic abuse surveillance as an early prevention tool for antimicrobial resistance. ECS J Solid State Sci Technol [Internet] [cited 2025 Aug 18];13(1):017003. Available from: https://iopscience.iop.org/article/10.1149/2162-8777/ad1c8d
9. Chaudhary V, Mostafavi E, Kaushik A (2022) De-coding Ag as an efficient antimicrobial nano-system for controlling cellular/biological functions. Matter [Internet] [cited 2025 Aug 18];5(7):1995–1998. Available from: https://www.cell.com/action/showFullText?pii=S2590238522003198
10. Taha BA, Ahmed NM, Talreja RK, Haider AJ, Al Mashhadany Y, Al-Jubouri Q et al (2024) Synergizing nanomaterials and artificial intelligence in advanced optical biosensors for precision antimicrobial resistance diagnosis. ACS Synth Biol [Internet] [cited 2025 Aug 18];13(6):1600–1620. Available from: https://pubs.acs.org/doi/abs/10.1021/acssynbio.4c00070
11. Kaur I, Priya N, Kumari A, Chaudhary V, Batra V (2022) Comprehensive study on indian plant extracts mediated biocompatible ZnO nanostructures: a green initiative. ECS Trans [Internet] [cited 2024 May 25];107(1):19443–19452. Available from: https://iopscience.iop.org/article/10.1149/10701.19443ecst
12. Mathur M, Verma A, Singh A, Yadav BC, Chaudhary V (2023) CuMoO4 nanorods-based acetone chemiresistor-enabled non-invasive breathomic-diagnosis of human diabetes and environmental monitoring. Environ Res [Internet] [cited 2025 Aug 18];229:115931. Available from: https://www.sciencedirect.com/science/article/abs/pii/S0013935123007235
13. Sable H, Kumar V, Singh V, Rustagi S, Chahal S, Chaudhary V (2024) Strategically engineering advanced nanomaterials for heavy-metal remediation from wastewater. Coord Chem Rev [Internet] [cited 2024 Jul 26];518:216079. Available from: https://linkinghub.elsevier.com/retrieve/pii/S0010854524004259
14. Antonacci A, Arduini F, Moscone D, Palleschi G, Scognamiglio V (2018) Nanostructured (bio)sensors for smart agriculture. TrAC- Trends Anal Chem 98:95–103
15. Panayi E, Peters GW, Kyriakides G (2017) Statistical modelling for precision agriculture: a case study in optimal environmental schedules for Agaricus Bisporus production via variable domain functional regression. PLoS One [Internet] [cited 2025 Jun 7];12(9):e0181921. Available from: https://journals.plos.org/plosone/article?id=10.1371/journal.pone.0181921
16. Sable H, Singh V, Kumar V, Roy A, Pandit S, Kaur K et al (2024) Toxicological and bioremediation profiling of nonessential heavy metals (mercury, chromium, cadmium, aluminium) and their impact on human health: a review. Toxicologie Analytique et Clinique [Internet]; Available from: https://linkinghub.elsevier.com/retrieve/pii/S2352007824001185

17. Chaudhary V, Bhadola P, Kaushik A, Khalid M, Furukawa H, Khosla A (2022) Assessing temporal correlation in environmental risk factors to design efficient area-specific COVID-19 regulations: Delhi based case study. Sci Rep [Internet] [cited 2025 Feb 14];12(1):1–16. Available from: https://www.nature.com/articles/s41598-022-16781-4
18. Larsson DGJ, Flach CF (2021) Antibiotic resistance in the environment. Nat Rev Microbiol [Internet] [cited 2025 Feb 2];20(5):257–269. Available from: https://www.nature.com/articles/s41579-021-00649-x
19. Raghavendra G, Mahija D, Sreevani T, Yamala A, Bindu PH (2017) Cell viability studies of green synthesised ZnO nanoparticles for antibacterial properties. Am J Mater Synth Process [Internet] [cited 2024 May 29];2(5):56–60. Available from: https://www.sciencepg.com/article/10.11648/j.ajmsp.20170205.11
20. John Sushma N, Prathyusha D, Swathi G, Madhavi T, Deva Prasad Raju B, Mallikarjuna K et al (2016) Facile approach to synthesize magnesium oxide nanoparticles by using Clitoria ternatea—characterization and in vitro antioxidant studies. Appl Nanosci (Switzerland) [Internet] [cited 2024 May 24];6(3):437–444. Available from: https://link.springer.com/article/10.1007/s13204-015-0455-1
21. Moradi G, Rahimi M, Zinadini S (2021) Antifouling nanofiltration membrane via tetrathioterephthalate coating on aniline oligomers-grafted polyethersulfone for efficient dye and heavy metal ion removal. J Environ Chem Eng 9(1):104717
22. Ciğeroğlu Z, El Messaoudi N, Şenol ZM, Başkan G, Georgin J, Gubernat S (2024) Clay-based nanomaterials and their adsorptive removal efficiency for dyes and antibiotics: a review. Mater Today Sustain 26:100735
23. Bunu SJ, Otele D, Alade T, Dodoru R (2020) Determination of serum DNA purity among patients undergoing antiretroviral therapy using NanoDrop-1000 spectrophotometer and polymerase chain reaction. Biomed Biotechnol Res J 4(3):214–219
24. Sun J, Warden AR, Huang J, Wang W, Ding X (2019) Colorimetric and electrochemical detection of Escherichia coli and antibiotic resistance based on a p-Benzoquinone-mediated bioassay. Anal Chem [Internet] [cited 2025 Jan 7];91(12):7524–7530. Available from: https://pubmed.ncbi.nlm.nih.gov/31117398/
25. Chaudhary V, Rustagi S et al (2024 undefined) Perspective—prospect of nano-enabled optical biosensors for antibiotic abuse surveillance as an early prevention tool for antimicrobial resistance. iopscience.iop.org [Internet] [cited 2025 Jan 7]; Available from: https://iopscience.iop.org/article/10.1149/2162-8777/ad1c8d/meta
26. Anjum M, Schmitt H et al (2021 undefined) The potential of using E. coli as an indicator for the surveillance of antimicrobial resistance (AMR) in the environment. Elsevier [Internet] [cited 2025 Jan 7]; Available from: https://www.sciencedirect.com/science/article/pii/S1369527421001302
27. Nag P, Sadani K, Mukherji S, Mukherji S (2020) Beta-lactam antibiotics induced bacteriolysis on LSPR sensors for assessment of antimicrobial resistance and quantification of antibiotics. Sens Actuators B Chem 311:127945
28. Rani N, Yadav S, Mushtaq A, Rani S, Saini M, Rawat S et al (2024) Azadirachta indica peel extract-mediated synthesis of ZnO nanoparticles for antimicrobial, supercapacitor and photocatalytic applications. Chem Papers [Internet] [cited 2024 May 29];78(6):3687–3704. Available from: https://link.springer.com/article/10.1007/s11696-024-03340-6
29. Devadas S, Zakaria Z, Shariff M, Bhassu S, Aquaculture MK (2023 undefined) Methodologies and standards for monitoring antimicrobial use and antimicrobial resistance in shrimp aquaculture. Elsevier [Internet] [cited 2025 Jan 7]; Available from: https://www.sciencedirect.com/science/article/pii/S0044848623009900
30. Ramzan M, Raza A et al (2024 undefined) Detection of antimicrobial resistance (AMR) and antimicrobial susceptibility testing (AST) using advanced spectroscopic techniques: a review. Elsevier [Internet] [cited 2025 Jan 7]; Available from: https://www.sciencedirect.com/science/article/pii/S016599362400044X

31. Kaprou GD, Bergšpica I, Alexa EA, Alvarez-Ordóñez A, Prieto M (2021) Rapid methods for antimicrobial resistance diagnostics. mdpi.com [Internet] [cited 2025 Jan 7]; Available from: https://www.mdpi.com/2079-6382/10/2/209
32. Aarestrup FM, Woolhouse MEJ (2020) Using sewage for surveillance of antimicrobial resistance. Science (1979) 367(6478):630–632
33. Singh V, Kasana E, Batra J, Sable H, Saxena R (2022) Antimicrobial resistance: mechanisms, screening techniques and biosensors. J Pharm Negat Results [Internet] [cited 2025 Aug 18];13:1724–1735. Available from: https://pnrjournal.com/index.php/home/article/view/2049

3 Wastewater Surveillance: Monitoring Antibiotic Abuse

Harsh Sable, Vandana Singh, Mahesh Narayan,
Aashi Sable, and Muhammad Shafiq

3.1 Introduction

Antimicrobials and antibacterials serve as vital agents utilized in therapeutic management of healthcare, livestock husbandry, agricultural production, and various industries (Fig. 3.1). In recent decades, the issue of antimicrobial resistance (AMR) has garnered significant attention due to the profound effects that resistant microorganisms exert on health of public [1–3]. The issue of antibiotic pollution is increasingly concerning, as it arises from the release of antibiotics into the environment, posing risks to organisms and facilitating the development of antibiotic resistance (Fig. 3.2). As a result, this has been identified as a significant issue for health of public worldwide.

H. Sable
Department of Forensic Science, School of Life and Applied Sciences, Maya Devi University, Dehradun, Uttarakhand, India

V. Singh (✉)
Department of Microbiology, Sharda School of Allied Health Sciences, Sharda University, Greater Noida, UP, India
e-mail: vandana.singh@sharda.ac.in

M. Narayan
Department of Chemistry and Biochemistry, The University of Texas at El Paso, El Paso, TX, USA

A. Sable
University of Kassel, Witzenhausen, Germany

Hochschule Fulda, University of Applied Sciences, Fulda, Germany

M. Shafiq
Research Institute of Clinical Pharmacy, Department of Pharmacology, Shantou University Medical College, Guangdong, China

V. Chaudhary, N. Bhalla (eds.), *Biosensors for Tackling Antimicrobial Resistance (AMR)*, https://doi.org/10.1007/978-981-95-9151-0_3

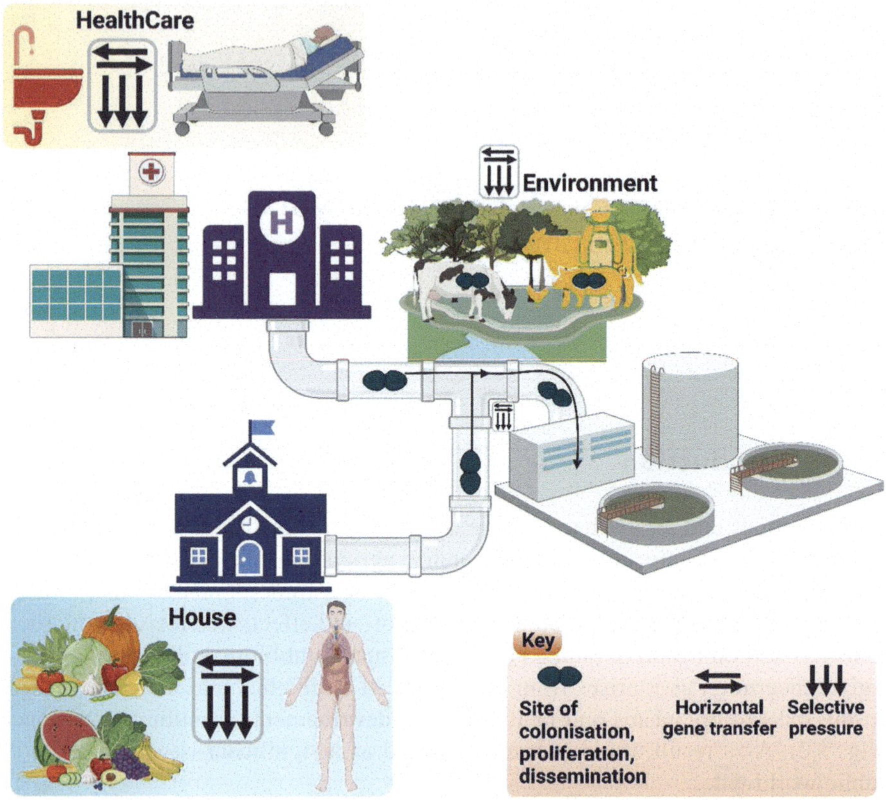

Fig. 3.1 Origins of antibiotic-resistant bacteria (ARBs) and antibiotic-resistant genes (ARGs) in wastewater. ARBs are present in humans, food, animals, agriculture, pipes, and sinks, ultimately entering wastewater. In wastewater, ARGs can be transferred between bacteria through horizontal gene transfer

The WHO (World Health Organization) defines antimicrobial resistance as a phenomenon where bacteria evolve and proliferate despite the existence of an antimicrobial (AM) agent. This phenomenon occurs when microorganisms, such as viruses, fungi, parasites, and bacteria, become unaffected by an antimicrobial agent to which they were once sensitive. This change is due to mutations in the microorganisms allow them to evade the effects of antimicrobials, or the resistance genes acquisition. By the year 2050, projections indicate that the number of human fatalities associated with AMR could reach ten million, leading to an economic burden of approximately $100 billion. While there is strong economic rationale for advancing antibiotics newer generations by the year 2030, the rate at which resistance to newer drug is emerging has become a critical factor in their potential introduction [4–6].

WHO established an array of AMs, specifically ABs (antibiotics), that are significant in both medicine for humans and animal medicine. The primary antimicrobials include macrolides, ketolides, and polymyxins, quinolones, and glycopeptides.

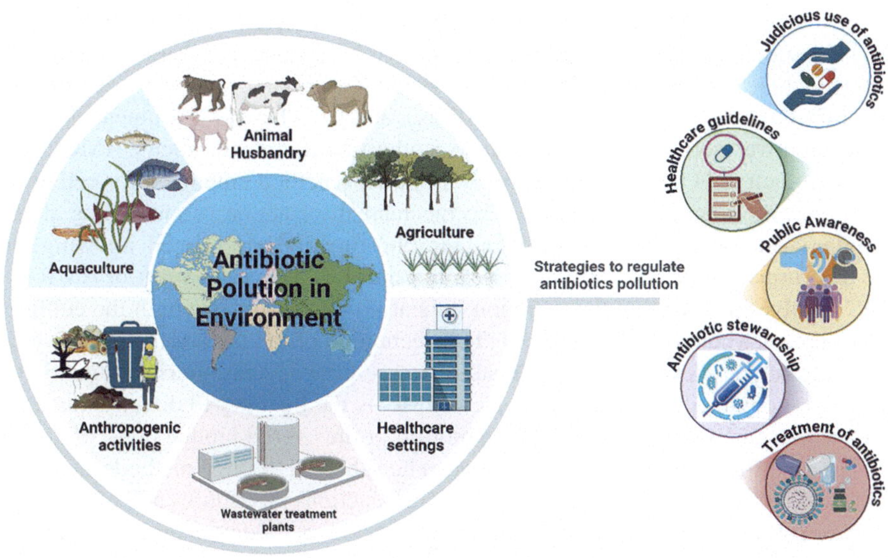

Fig. 3.2 The sources and implications of antibiotic contamination. Strategies to reduce the pollution caused by antibiotics

The WHO, in the year 2017 released a list of antibiotic-resistant pathogens, identifying 12 families of bacteria prioritized for discovering and developing new ABs. This initiative addresses the increasing demand for novel treatments targeting bacteria which are multi-resistant in health care facilities. The empirical application of broad-ranging antimicrobials in veterinary and clinical practices is a primary factor contributing to the global rise in antimicrobial resistance. Early detection of microorganisms is crucial for disease prevention and the control of AMR. Therefore, it is essential to establish laboratories which are well-equipped, that specialize in infection diagnosis. Meeting this requirement in developing countries is challenging due to insufficient funding, a shortage of trained personnel, and inadequate infrastructure. The EUCAST (European Committee on Antimicrobial Susceptibility Testing) guidelines stipulate that dependable AMR tests necessitate phenotypic evaluation, which involves experimental processes to assess growth of microbe in the presence of antimicrobials. The standard procedure for assessing pathogen resistance involves isolation techniques, such as enrichment culture (e.g., Culture of urine) and cultivation on plates, followed by identification, and AST (antimicrobial susceptibility testing) utilizing various antimicrobial load. The findings can be articulated as the minimal concentrations of the AB that inhibits visible growth, referred to as the MIC (minimal inhibitory concentration). ASTs utilizing methods of culturing necessitate a duration of 24–72 h. This lapse of time may be critical for the patient. A further limitation of culture-based techniques is the necessity for trained personnel. The test of disk diffusion, introduced by Bauer and Kirby in the 1960 to assess antibiotic susceptibility in *Staphylococcus* strains, remains one of the most utilized phenotypic methods for AST. The assays for broth microdilution represent a widely utilized technique that relies on visible growth. Commercially available automated AST instruments have decreased analysis times to under one day. Automated instruments include the MicroScan WalkAway system (Beckman Coulter), Vitek systems (BioMèrieux), Alfred 60AST system (Alifax), and BD Phoenix instruments [4, 7].

Alternative methods for AST include isothermal microcalorimetry (IMC) and flow cytometry (FC). Flow cytometry is an optical method employed for cell enumeration and biomarker detection. The mechanism of action of antibiotics alters certain physiological characteristics and morpho-functional of the cell, allowing for the determination of susceptibility levels through FC. The assessment of AMR by IMC involves quantifying the variation in heat production rates within the cultural environment when an AM is present. This technique offers the advantage of being non-destructive. Nevertheless, the results may require several hours or potentially days to be obtained. Another downside of IMC is the inability to directly quantify cells which cannot replicate within the biofilm or the overall biomass [7–10].

The identification of resistance genes can be achieved through methods based on nucleic acids, such as PCR (polymerase chain reaction) procedures and other technologies of amplification of nucleic acid. Genotypic methods are limited to identifying specific resistances, as they evaluate only selected genes. Furthermore, DNA extraction is essential as complex matrices can result in significant interpretation challenges; thus, the resistance genes identified may not originate from the pathogen itself. The method based on PCR may yield unspecific results if the primer is inadequately designed or misaligned with other DNA regions, leading to false positives. The WGS (whole-genome sequencing) of the utilizing pathogen NGS (next generation sequencing) offers a comprehensive overview of the resistome of pathogen, including the prediction of known resistance phenotypes. Nonetheless, similarly to PCR, this technique does not demonstrate the potential functionality of the microorganism's genes. The resolution of this issue can be achieved through metagenomics that is functional; however, it requires an extended duration due to the insertion of target genes into a plasmid, which are then introduced into a host, such as strain of bacteria [9]. This is followed by the AST and culturing process, contributing to the overall time required. Microarray technology and FISH (fluorescence in situ hybridization) are commonly employed techniques for evaluating gene resistance, utilizing various synthetic capture probes, including (peptide nucleic acid) PNA probes. Though, the development of PNA-FISH typically involves prior culture of biological samples using automated instruments, which extends the analysis time [11–13].

3.2 Biosensors and Sensors for AMR Detection

The effectiveness of biosensors in identifying AMR in wastewater relies on their ability to utilize minimal reagent and sample volumes, ensuring high detection capacity even at low nano concentration levels. Biological integration enables the use of receptors for molecules, DNA, or antibodies as components of biorecognition. They may also operate by means of interference or the consideration of enzyme-analyte interactions. Biosensor and chemosensor technologies represent an alternate method characterized by cost effective and technological simplicity, reduced time of analysis, and ease of operation. These technologies show significant potential for delivering essential information for concurrent collection of data and analysis in real time evaluation of various analytes within one apparatus. Chemosensors quantify the signal generated by a reaction of chemicals. In contrast, Biosensors are compacted instruments for analysis that integrate a biologically derived or biological sensing element with a physicochemical transducer, either within the device or in close association with it [14–18].

Various biosensors for AST and detection of resistance gene have been documented in the literature. Real matrices which are complex have been examined, encompassing biological matrices like blood, urine, and saliva, as well as environmental matrices including soil, various water sources, vegetation, domestic animals, and foodstuff. Sensors differ from bioassays and bioanalytical systems in that they do not typically necessitate multiple additional steps involving reagent addition. However, certain bioassays can be advanced into biosensors through process automation. Biosensors possess significant advantages over conventional methods and batch systems, including high detection capacity, cost-effective automation, and easy to operate automated (robotic) analytical procedures. Biosensors utilize immobilization materials and techniques to enhance the stability of their biomolecular components [19–21]. This chapter aims to describe techniques for detecting AMR that are based on sensors and biosensors, focusing specifically on systems proposed for genotypic and phenotypic AMR detection. Consequently, methods based on biosensors for the identification of general pathogens are not included in this review.

3.3 Commercial Antibiotic Detection Sensors

Detection of antibiotic residues is crucial for ensuring water safety, environmental monitoring, and clinical diagnostics. This chapter primarily presents commercially available technologies for detecting antibiotics in various sample types, followed by a discussion on recently introduced biosensors and devices. Numerous commercially accessible sensors are being designed to meet this need, providing different detection mechanisms and varying levels of specificity, practicality, and sensitivity. This section examines four primary groups of technologies for antibiotic detection: (a) gold-standard technologies, (b) Nano-based sensors, (c) emerging electrochemical-based biosensors and devices, and (d) optical-based sensors.

3.3.1 Gold-Standard Technologies

Gold-standard technology refers to a method that has undergone extensive testing and has demonstrated high reliability. Effective methods for detecting antibiotics in various samples include traditional techniques such as HPLC (high-performance liquid chromatography), (UV–Vis) ultraviolet–visible spectroscopy, CE (capillary electrophoresis), MS (mass spectrometry), and microbiological assays, which are valued for their sensitivity, reliability, and accuracy. HPLC coupled with MS is recognized for its accuracy in antibiotic detection. The Infinity II LC 1290 system from Agilent delivers high resolution and efficiency, whereas Thermo Fisher's TSQ Quantis MS enables precise quantification of ABs at extremely low concentrations (ppb). Microbiological assays represent a significant technology, recognized for their capacity to identify a broad spectrum of antibiotics via inhibition of growth of microbes. Neogen Corporation, located in Lansing, USA, and Charm Sciences, based in Lawrence, USA, are prominent suppliers in this field. CE is a reliable method for the analysis of ABs. Sciex, based in Framingham, MA, USA, has launched the Pharmaceutical Analysis System PA 800 Plus. This system enables quantification of Abs and high-resolution separation across diverse samples, achieving Low detection limits (ng mL^{-1}). UV–Vis spectroscopy is a traditional method employed for the purpose of antibiotic detection. In the recent decades, numerous companies have launched significant technologies and products aimed at detecting ABs in various samples. Table 3.1 summarizes several examples along with their associated working parameters [22–26].

The traditional approaches, supported by products from prominent companies, yield extremely sensitive, precise, and repeatable outcomes, rendering them crucial in identifying and monitoring antibiotic residues in various samples. Despite their outstanding capabilities, the portability and cost of such technologies present major barriers, especially in situations with limited resources where access to advanced funding, and equipment is restricted. The budget constrains and the cumbersome characteristics of these devices restrict their broad practicality and application in these contexts. Consequently, engineers and scientists are investigating design methodologies, innovative materials, and production methods to develop future technologies that are both highly portable and cost-effective. This facilitates the broader installation of critical diagnostic tools, addressing the diverse requirements of countless applications and geographical regions, thereby enhancing effectiveness and accessibility [22, 24].

Table 3.1 Table of exemplary gold-standard methods for antibiotic detection, including analysis duration

Company	Technology	Product	LoD	Time required	Reference
ThermoFisher Scientific	HPLC and MS	Vanquish UHPLC and Orbitrap MS	Ppb levels	30–60 min per sample	[27, 28]
Charm Sciences	Microbiological assays	ROSA Lateral Flow System	Low ppb levels	1–2 h per batch	[29]
Sciex	CE	Capillary Electrophoresis System	Low ng/ml range	Per sample 20–40 min	[30]
Waters Corporation	LC-MS/UV-Vis	Xevo TQ-S micro LC-MS/MS System	Ppt levels	Per sample 30–60 min	[31]

3.3.2 Nano-based Sensors

Nanobiosensors are efficient and cost-effective devices for this application. A nanobiosensor refers to a type of biosensor that utilizes nanoparticles in its construction to detect specific chemical, or biological substances. These sensors integrate an element for biological recognition, including enzyme, nucleic acids, or antibodies, with a transducer such as optical, electrical, and mechanical that converts the interaction among the material of target and recognizing the element in a quantifiable signal. Nanomaterials employed in biosensors, including nanowires, nanoparticles, and graphene, facilitate improved specificity, sensitivity, and detection speed owing to their substantial ratio of volume to surface area, and distinctive characteristics. Nano biosensors primarily function to detect biologically specific materials and facilitate monitoring of water and environmental. These materials typically include antibodies, proteins, enzymes, and biomolecules. Nanobiosensors are employed for the direct detection of pollutants and microbes for monitoring of environment and wastewater [32–35].

In the research conducted by Inbaraj and Chen (2016) to identify aquatic E. coli, "The E. coli O157:H7 eaeA gene was targeted using a thiolated DNA (single-stranded) probe that self-assembled onto the QCM sensor." The subsequent stages included the induction of hybridization by exposing the (single-stranded) DNA probe to the target DNA that is complementary and amplifying it by primers that are biotin-labelled for asymmetric PCR. This led to a variation in mass accompanied by a corresponding alteration in QCM frequency for the identification of O157:H7 E. coli. The determined detection limit was 2.67×10^2 CFU/mL [36].

The work by Margo et al. (2022) on mineral water revealed that TiO_2 and ZnO based sensors, fabricated using DC magnetron sputtering with either 50% or 100% O_2 in the sputtering chamber, successfully detected three macrolides at ranging concentrations from 10^{-5} to 10^{-15} M. The PCA analysis of river water revealed distinct patterns and trends differentiating between doped and non-doped samples, as well as categorizing various amounts of azithromycin, clarithromycin, and erythromycin. Utilizing the e-tongue concept with both matrices, sensitivity values of 4.6 ± 0.3, 4.8 ± 0.3, and 4.5 ± 0.3 per decade were obtained for azithromycin, erythromycin, and clarithromycin, concentrations, respectively. A resolution of 1×10^{-16} M was seen around the 10^{-15} M concentrations, which was the lowermost AB concentrations recorded in all instances [37].

In the investigation by Li and Sun 2021, graphene dispersion was used to co-mingle with E. coli cells to enhance the current signal. This electrochemical sensor facilitates the assessment of E. coli activity on the surface of electrode. The presence of antibiotics attenuated the electrocatalytic reduction signal due to the decreased activity of E. coli. The variation in the electrochemical reduction signal allows for the assessment of antibiotic resistance among various E. coli strains [38].

Gwyther, 2024, employed sophisticated sampling techniques in conjunction with not-canonical amino acid chemistry to model the electrostatic potential of proteins on (SWCNTs) single-walled carbon nanotubes. The study centers on (BLIP2) β-lactamase binding protein as the receptor, which interacts with antibiotic-degrading enzymes known as (BLs) β-lactamases. BLIP2 is covalently linked to SWCNTs through a genetically encoded phenyl azide photochemistry at a singular selected residue. The devices developed are capable of detecting two distinct TEM-1, KPC-2, and BLs, each producing unique conductance profiles attributable to their varying surface electrostatic characteristics [39].

3.3.3 Optical-Based Sensors

Optical biosensors are the predominant category of biosensors used in commercial applications. Use of optical biosensors for analyte detection relies on the interactions between a biorecognition component and an optical field. Optical biosensors may be catalogued into two categories: label-free and label-based. Label-free biosensors produce an electrical signal immediately from the contact between the analyte and the transducer. An instance of this is biosensors based on surface plasmon resonance (SPR) which are optical, which are used for detecting pathogens in both water and food. In contrast, Label-based sensing depends on a label, resulting in the optical signal typically produced by a luminescent, fluorescent, or colorimetric response. Colorimetric sensors present several advantages, such as an easy process, inexpensiveness, and the capability to detect colour changes either visually or through basic instrumentation for analysing data quantitatively. Chemical species that exhibit colour changes in response to bacterial growth, like Resazurin, and enzymes such as Horseradish Peroxidase (HRP), which alter substrates based on microbial cell counts, facilitate real-time measurement of susceptibility [15, 40–43].

In the study conducted by Sun et al., p-benzoquinone served as a tool to assess bacterial concentration and effectively differentiate *E. coli* from four other prevalent bacterial species: *Staphylococcus aureus*, *Enterococcus faecalis*, *Salmonella pullorum*, and *Streptococcus mutans*. A noticeable colour shift, assessed without sophisticated equipment but with just a basic smartphone, is employed to ascertain the concentration of bacteria [44].

Numerous kinds of biosensors utilize labels which are fluorescent, including nanomaterials. Nazemi et al. devised a swift method for assessing the E. Coli antibiotic susceptibility using GaAs/AlGaAs quantum well (QW) biochips' photoluminescence (PL) emission. Bacterium cells were immobilized on the surface of quantum well, resulting in a delay of a maximum photoluminescence. The biochips were made functional using polyclonal antibodies specific to *E. Coli*. Following a 4-h incubation in LB broth, ciprofloxacin, or penicillin, the position of the maximum photoluminescence was assessed. The maximum PL is influenced by the process of photocorrosion resulting from the GaAs/AlGaAs biochips' surface contains immobilized microorganisms (Fig. 3.3a). Antibiotic exposure accelerates peak photoluminescence in bacterial cells compared to their presence in LB medium [45].

Tang et al. investigated the changes in resultant pH resulting from the rapid buildup of metabolic byproducts from cellular development. This work produced combining poly(dimethylsiloxane) microfluidic channels with pH-sensitive chitosan hydrogel to create a microfluidic pH sensor. Fourier transform reflectometric

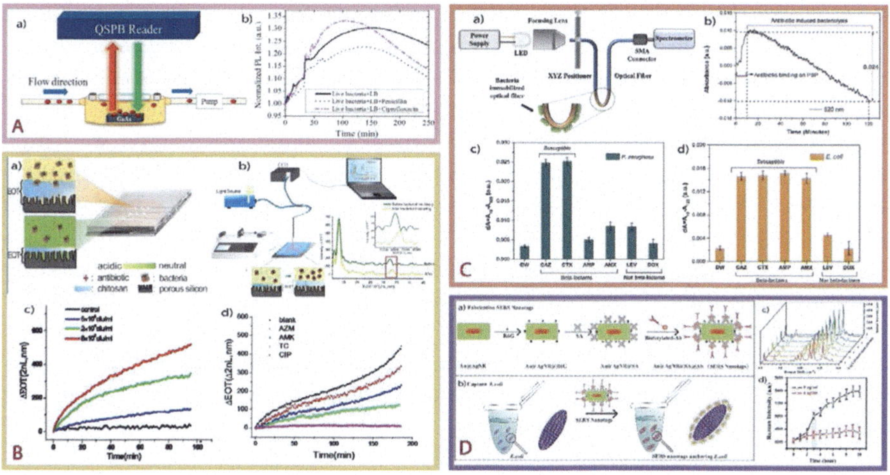

Fig. 3.3 Various optical biosensors utilized for antimicrobial susceptibility testing (AST) are presented. (**a**) (a) Schematic representation of the experimental configuration; (b) normalized photoluminescence intensity recorded for biochips in E. coli subjected to penicillin and ciprofloxacin. Adapted from Ref. [45], Copyright, 2017 Elsevier, 6111250888576. (**b**) (a) Mechanism for monitoring bacterial metabolism and growth; (b) schematic of the instrumental setup for sample detection; (c) time traces of EOT changes during bacterial incubation in the microfluidic channel; (d) EOT changes measured by the sensor containing bacteria with varying concentrations of antibiotics. Adapted from Ref. [46]. Copyright, 2013 American Chemical Society, 6111251193916. (**c**) (a) Optical detection assembly; (b) time-varying response of P. aeruginosa immobilized optical fibers to 10 µg/mL ceftazidime; (c) response of P. aeruginosa; and (d) E. coli immobilized optical fiber to 10 µg/mL of antibiotics. DW represents the variation in absorbance observed in distilled water alone. Adapted from Ref. [47], Copyright, 2020 Elsevier, 6111251499521. (**d**) (a) Diagram illustrating the functionalization process of Au@AgNR as a SERS nanotag; (b) binding of the SERS nanotag to E. coli; (c) SERS spectra of the E. coli complex at varying concentrations from 10^7 to 10^2 CFU/mL; (d) growth curve of E. coli derived from SERS data following exposure to ampicillin (4 µg/mL) and in the absence of exposure. (Adapted from Ref. [48], Copyright, 2020 Elsevier, 6111260421569)

interference spectroscopy (FTIR) was employed to monitor the change in pH. The cells of bacteria (1×10^6 CFU/mL, *E. coli*) suspended with various ABs (tetracycline, ciprofloxacin, amikacin, and azithromycin) were inserted into the device for reflectance spectra measurement. Increased EOT was assessed in actual time by evaluating the potential hindering of the growth of bacteria by various antibiotics (Fig. 3.3b). This method effectively monitored the growth of microbes and the MIC of antibiotics in actual time, specifically amikacin at 16 µg/mL, azithromycin at 1 µg/mL, tetracycline at 0.5 µg/mL, and ciprofloxacin at 0.25 µg/mL, within a 60-min timeframe [46].

Nag et al.'s work showed that a rapid analysis of antibiotic susceptibility (doxycycline, amoxicillin, ceftazidime, ampicillin, cefotaxime, and levofloxacin) in *E. coli* and *P. aeruginosa* gold nanoparticles and localized SPR are used. The analysis involved the direct capture of bacteria (10^5 CFU/mL) from urine using an optical fiber sensor coated with gold nanoparticles (Fig. 3.3c). Following this, the bacteria were subjected to cell lysis using various antibiotics for a duration of 2 h, during which the changes in absorbance were monitored to assess the resistance or susceptibility of the bacteria to the different ABs (Fig. 3.3c). The sensor was additionally evaluated using drinking water specimens [47].

Au@AgNR nanorods with a core-shell structure that are SERS-active were used by Bi et al. to create an AST process. As shown in Fig. 3.3d, the SERS nanotag system was created by functionalizing Au@AgNR with (SA) streptavidin and then interacting with biotinylated antibodies unique to E. coli to generate full SERS nanotags (Au@AgNR@SA@Ab). The biosensor's sensitivity was evaluated by capturing bacterial cells with nanotags (Fig. 3.3d) and assessing them at different CFU concentrations. The susceptibility of the bacterial cells was then evaluated by exposing them to ampicillin. The technique demonstrated 10^2 CFU/mL as the detection limit, an analysis time estimated of less than 4 h, and the capability to analyses matrices of biology, including blood [48].

3.3.4 Electrochemical- Based Biosensor

Electrochemical biosensors are used in water safety, monitoring of environment, and industrial/medical diagnosis. Four elements make up these sensors: (a) a recognition element that selectively interacts with the molecule of target, (b) a transducer that converts the signal into a measurable output, (c) an electrolyte for electrochemical reactions, and (d) electrodes (reference, counter, and work). Figure 3.4a illustrates the operating principle of an electrochemical biosensor. Current electrochemical biosensors include potentiometric, amperometric, and impedimetric forms (Fig. 3.4b).

Electrochemical sensors are being considered for application in AST tests. Electroactive bacteria are capable of performing a diverse range of the redox reactions. Electrochemical sensors effectively assess the electrical responses of cells of bacteria with high sensitivity, often bypassing extended isolation and culturing periods, enabling direct measurement in biological and environmental matrices. The response can be measured either directly, or indirectly, contingent upon the interaction between the bacteriological cell and the element of recognition. In direct detection, the interaction between the cell and an immobilized bacteriophage or antibody on the electrode results in a change in electron transfer, influenced by the activity of membrane enzymes. The cell is induced to release electroactive chemicals that may be measured via indirect detection [49–52].

Hannah et al. developed a solid-phase extraction (SPE) method to monitor growth of the bacteria and identify the appropriate antibiotic for treating *E. coli* infections, facilitating low-cost diagnostics. Using electrochemical impedance spectroscopy (EIS), an antibiotic-seeded hydrogel was used to modify a gold electrode and determine the E. coli strains' resistance to current flow. After 2.5 h of exposure to 4 μg/mL of streptomycin (MIC), the bacteria showed a sensitivity of 10^5 CFU/mL [53]. Table 3.2 presents various electrochemical sensors that have been developed over the past decade, along with the different identification components employed to assess antimicrobial susceptibility.

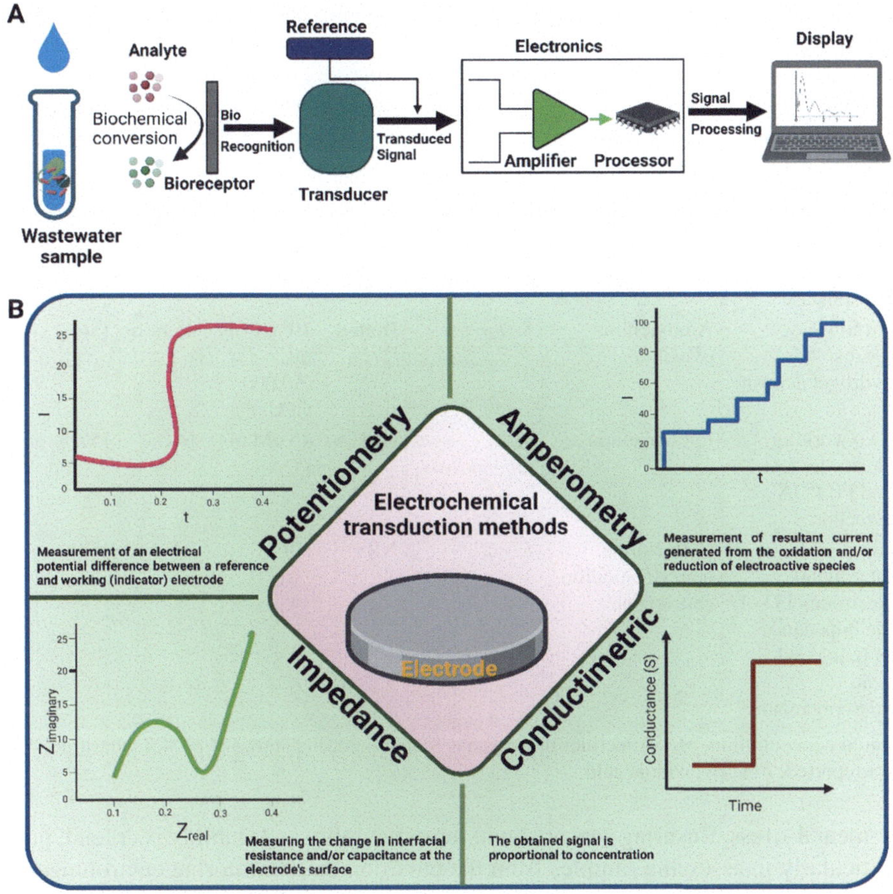

Fig. 3.4 Diagrammatic illustration of (**a**) a generic biosensor device demonstrating the target's interaction with the bioreceptor in a sample. The transducer is in charge of producing a signal following recognition. (**b**) Electrochemical transduction signal examples

3.4 Challenges Related to Biosensors in AMR Detection

- **Variable and Complex Wastewater Matrices**: Wastewater comprises a diverse mixture of inorganic as well as organic compounds, toxic metals, bacteria, and other contaminants. These components of the matrix may disrupt biosensor performance by inducing non-specific binding, fouling sensor surfaces, and suppressing signals. The variability in the pH level, temperature, and turbidity exacerbates the repeatability and sensitivity of biosensor experiments [59].
- **Durability and Stability**: Wastewater biosensors degrade and lose functionality due to severe chemical and biological conditions. Nucleic acids, enzymes, and antibodies immobilized on sensor surfaces are especially susceptible to environ-

Table 3.2 Electrochemical biosensor for determining antimicrobial susceptibility

Electrode-recognizing element	Antibiotic	Target	MIC (μg/L)	Limit of detection	Time	Reference
SPE-Thiolated oligonucleotide capture probes	Ciprofloxacin	*E. coli*	2	10^3 CFU/mL	5 h	[54]
Au SPE-antibody alkaline phosphatase	MRSA strain	*S. aureus*	Nm	845 CFU/mL	4.5 h	[55]
Au SPE-agarose-based hydrogel deposit	Amoxicillin, oxacillin	*S. aureus*	Both 8	10^7 CFU/mL (50,000 CFUs)[a]	45 min	[56]
Two working electrodes (Au and Pt) POA detection	Pyrazinamide	*M. tuberculosis*	NM	40 uM of POA	NR	[57]
Array of interdigital electrodes-FD of the impedance of living and dead microorganisms	Ceftazidime, benzylpenicillin, ceftriaxone	*E. coli*	NR	NR	2 h	[58]

[a]Initial concentration, *MRSA* methicillin-resistant Staphylococcus aureus, *NM* Not measured, *NR* Not reported, *POA* pyrazinoic acid

mental stress. Ensuring sensor signal reproducibility and stability is crucial, particularly in assessing samples from the environment. Monitoring environmental analytes on the spot is more challenging than experimenting with artificial specimens owing to the complex air, water, and soil environment (e.g., inorganic, and organic chemicals, turbidity, pH). It is challenging to identify many environmental contaminants (Fig. 3.5) [60, 61].

- **Lack of Standardization and Calibration Protocols**: The lack of standard procedures for the calibration, validation, and interpretation of data from biosensors is a barrier to their broad adoption. The discrepancies that are found across various research are caused by differences in the detection procedures and the interpretation of the findings.
- **Low Abundance of AMR Markers**: Resistant bacterial strains and AMR genes often exist in low quantities inside wastewater, complicating their identification. Contemporary biosensors may exhibit insufficient sensitivity to identify trace quantities of AMR biomarkers without pre-concentration or amplification procedures. Producing electrochemical sensors capable of detecting analytes at varying concentrations, with low limits of detection and high stability, remains challenging. The sensitivity of traditional electrodes (e.g., gold) is often constrained by their slower redox kinetics. Further investigation is required to provide cost-effective and extremely stable electrode materials for extreme conditions [59].

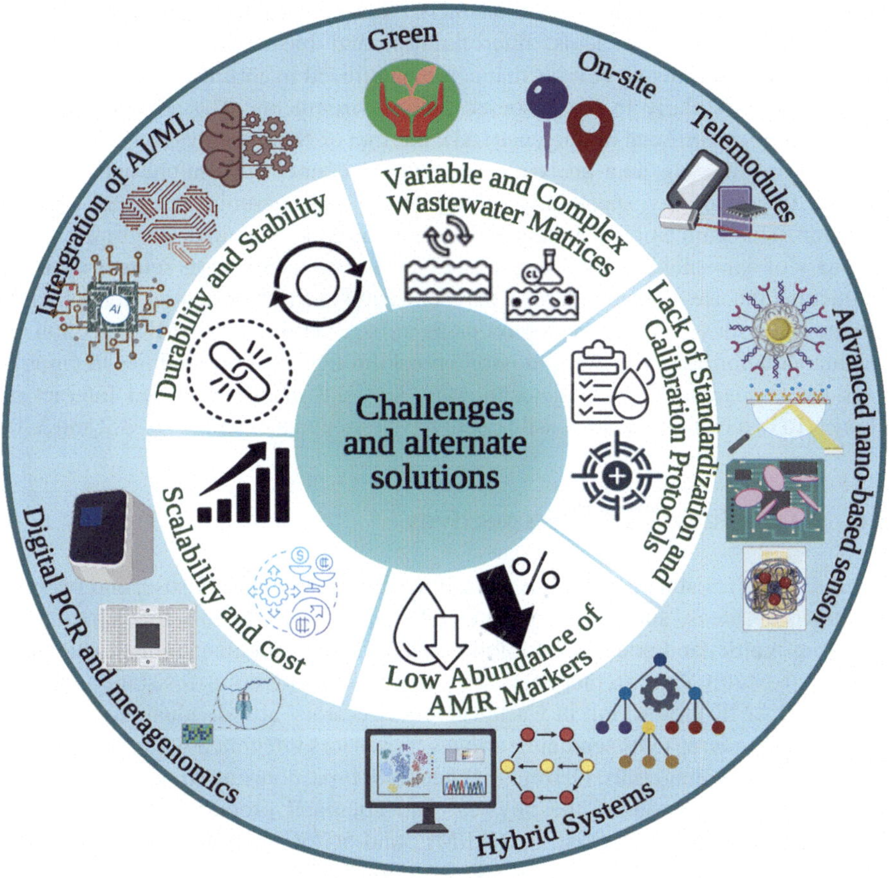

Fig. 3.5 Biosensor for wastewater monitoring of antibiotic misuse, challenges, alternative solutions: a pathway to early detection and prevention of AMR

- **Scalability and cost**: The higher cost may restrict the extensive use of these sensors, especially in resource-limited environments where financial limitations are a critical issue. Consequently, while the inexpensiveness of biosensors is beneficial, more efforts are required to lower expenses and enhance the reliability and accessibility of these technologies for a wider audience.

3.5 Alternative Solutions

The application of biosensors will facilitate the creation of multiplexing formats for quick point-of-care devices [62]. Advancements in various transducing techniques will enable antimicrobial resistance monitoring without resources in low-source requiring trained personnel. Transducer miniaturization and their integration with microfluidic platforms will facilitate the development of user-friendly, compact, and multiplexed systems, thereby enhancing the acceptance of biosensors between industrial stakeholders and end consumers. Recent breakthroughs in isothermal amplification of nucleic acids, microfluidics, and biosensor technologies have yielded several promising devices that could be utilized in antimicrobial susceptibility testing, particularly in low-resource field environments. The amalgamation of nanotechnology, artificial intelligence (AI), Internet of Nano-Things (IoNT), sustainable engineering, big data analytics, and 5G/6G connectivity might substantially enhance the sensitivity, specificity, and rapidity of antimicrobial resistance (AMR) detection. This innovation is anticipated to transform the domain of diagnostics. The summary of nanoenabled AMR diagnostic biosensors encompasses sources of AMR production, the use of nanomaterials, the facilitation of fifth-generation technologies, and the categories of optical nanobiosensors utilized. Ultimately, AMR detection on a semiconductor presents several possible breakthroughs and possibilities. It emphasizes the amalgamation of nanotechnology, artificial intelligence, and Internet of Things (IoT) technologies as possible pathways for enhancement (Figs. 3.2 and 3.5).

3.6 Conclusion and Perspectives

Antimicrobial resistance (AMR) is caused by antibiotic abuse, misuse, and overuse in numerous areas, such as environmental management, healthcare, agriculture, industries, cattle, and poultry. Antibiotics (AB) threatens human, animal, and environmental health via carcinogenic, mutagenic, and microbial resistance effects. Therefore, AMR monitoring in wastewater is necessary at individual and community levels. Modern AMR screening utilizes biosensors integrated with optical, electrochemical, nanomaterials. Optimizing precursor type, concentration, and synthesis parameters may customize the physical and chemical properties of biosensors. Using current technologies like IoT, AI/ML, and 5G/6G communication networks may improve the effectiveness of AMR detection in these sensors. The merging of these technologies solves basic biosensor concerns and creates portability, smart, tailored, and remotely accessible modules. To address the potential for excessive solid waste from sensor use, consider using green biosensors and waste-to-wealth modules to promote a circular economy. Portable and tiny sensors help avoid antibiotic abuse in food production areas including agriculture and poultry farms. Furthermore, regulatory enforcers may utilize it as a wastewater monitoring tool to identify AMR in a neighbourhood. To combat AMR, smart nano-enabled optical biosensors can detect and prevent AB in certain circumstances. Modern biosensors may prevent AMR by detecting AB in wastewater, hospital, food production, industrial, and environmental contexts, potentially meeting UN sustainable development objectives. Biosensor devices are a promising technology for sensing due to their variety and ease of usage. These gadgets, known for their versatility, are increasingly viable options for medical diagnostics and environmental monitoring. Reliable and accurate measurements are essential for informed decision-making and public safety, addressing shortcomings with current gold-standard technology. Biosensors excel in providing accurate data quickly and effectively. These sensors may identify low-level contaminants in environmental monitoring, allowing prompt responses to avert ecological harm.

References

1. Singh V, Kasana E, Batra J, Sable H, Saxena R (2022) Antimicrobial resistance: mechanisms, screening techniques and biosensors. J Pharm Negat Results:1724–1735
2. Chaudhary V, Mostafavi E, Kaushik A (2022) De-coding Ag as an efficient antimicrobial nano-system for controlling cellular/biological functions. Matter 5:1995–1998
3. Pal A, Sable H, Uniyal A, Chaudhary V (2025) Green nano-semiconductors and nanometals to avert complex phenomena of antimicrobial resistance (AMR). Curr Opin Biomed Eng. https://doi.org/10.1016/j.cobme.2025.100626
4. Tacconelli E, Carrara E, Savoldi A et al (2018) Discovery, research, and development of new antibiotics: the WHO priority list of antibiotic-resistant bacteria and tuberculosis. Lancet Infect Dis 18:318–327
5. Hill R, Stentiford GD, Walker DI, Baker-Austin C, Ward G, Maskrey BH, Van Aerle R, Verner-Jeffreys D, Peeler E, Bass D. Realising a global One Health disease surveillance approach: insights from wastewater and beyond. https://doi.org/10.1038/s41467-024-49417-4
6. Murray CJ, Ikuta KS, Sharara F et al (2022) Global burden of bacterial antimicrobial resistance in 2019: a systematic analysis. Lancet 399:629–655
7. Reynoso EC, Laschi S, Palchetti I, Torres E (2021) Advances in antimicrobial resistance monitoring using sensors and biosensors: a review. Chemosensors 9:232
8. Rotilie CA, Fass RJ, Prior RB, Perkins RL (1975) Microdilution technique for antimicrobial susceptibility testing of anaerobic bacteria. Antimicrob Agents Chemother 7:311–315
9. Sable H, Vaishali, Singh V (2023) β2-microglobulin biomarkers' roles in assessing cadmium toxicity. Int J Med Toxicol Legal Med 26:112–116
10. Singh V, Sable H, Vaishali, Ghalley M, Tenzin K (2024) Environmental toxicology, fate and risk assessment of emerging contaminants. In: Occurrence, Distribution and Toxic Effects of Emerging Contaminantsx. CRC Press, pp 134–167
11. Li Y, Yang X, Zhao W (2017) Emerging microtechnologies and automated systems for rapid bacterial identification and antibiotic susceptibility testing. SLAS Technol 22:585–608
12. Dietvorst J, Vilaplana L, Uria N, Marco MP, Muñoz-Berbel X (2020) Current and near-future technologies for antibiotic susceptibility testing and resistant bacteria detection. TrAC- Trends Anal Chem. https://doi.org/10.1016/J.TRAC.2020.115891
13. Rani A, Kaur G, Kumar R, Sachan RSK, Kumar M, Sable H, Al Tawaha ARM, Malik S, Karnwal A, Malik T (2025) Role of DNA methylation in the pathogenesis of skin disorders: mechanisms, inhibitors of methylation-related enzyme, and molecular docking studies. Biomed Res Int 2025:7002918
14. Chaudhary V, Ahmed Taha B, Rustagi S, Khosla A, Papakonstantinou P, Bhalla N (2024) Nose-on-chip nanobiosensors for early detection of lung cancer breath biomarkers. ACS Publications. https://doi.org/10.1021/acssensors.4c01524
15. Taha BA, Ahmed NM, Talreja RK et al (2024) Synergizing nanomaterials and artificial intelligence in advanced optical biosensors for precision antimicrobial resistance diagnosis. ACS Synth Biol 13:1600–1620
16. Chauhan N, Sankhla MS, Sharma A, Sable H, Sharma T (2025) Nanotechnology-enhanced detection of illicit drugs: development of Nano sensors for rapid identification in liquid media. J Electrochem Soc 172:077505
17. Chaudhary V, Sable H, Kumar M, Prakash C, Sonu S (2025) Dynamic landscape of chemiresistive breathomic nanosensors based on fifth-generation chips for complex disease diagnosis and healthcare monitoring. Appl Phys Rev. https://doi.org/10.1063/5.0255483/3371043
18. Chaudhary V, Bhadola P (2025) Artificial intelligence-powered nanosensor platforms for non-invasive Breathomic diagnostics. Nanotechnol Sci Appl 18:611–641
19. Adator EH, Narvaez-Bravo C, Zaheer R, Cook SR, Tymensen L, Hannon SJ, Booker CW, Church D, Read RR, McAllister TA (2020) A one health comparative assessment of antimicrobial resistance in generic and extended-spectrum cephalosporin-resistant escherichia coli from beef production, sewage and clinical settings. Microorganisms 8:1–22

20. Michael CA, Dominey-Howes D, Labbate M (2014) The antimicrobial resistance crisis: causes, consequences, and management. Front Public Health. https://doi.org/10.3389/FPUBH.2014.00145
21. Chaudhary V, Lucky L, Sable H, Bhalla N (2025) Interdisciplinary approach to Monkeypox prevention: integrating nanobiosensors, nanovaccines, artificial intelligence, visual arts, and social sciences. Small Struct 6:2400647
22. Devadas S, Zakaria Z, Shariff M, Bhassu S, Aquaculture MK (2023 undefined) Methodologies and standards for monitoring antimicrobial use and antimicrobial resistance in shrimp aquaculture. Elsevier
23. Hassan S, Chemistry XZ-CA, 2020 undefined (2014) Microfluidics as an emerging platform for tackling antimicrobial resistance (AMR): a review. ingentaconnect.com 1
24. Salam M, Al-Amin M, Pawar J et al (2023 undefined) Conventional methods and future trends in antimicrobial susceptibility testing. Elsevier
25. Kaprou GD, Bergšpica I, Alexa EA, Alvarez-Ordóñez A, Prieto M (2021) Rapid methods for antimicrobial resistance diagnostics. mdpicom. https://doi.org/10.3390/antibiotics10020209
26. Ramzan M, Raza A et al (2024 undefined) Detection of antimicrobial resistance (AMR) and antimicrobial susceptibility testing (AST) using advanced spectroscopic techniques: a review. Elsevier
27. Vanquish HPLC and UHPLC Systems – IE
28. Vanquish HPLC and UHPLC Systems | Thermo Fisher Scientific – IE. https://www.thermofisher.com/ie/en/home/products-and-services/promotions/industrial/vanquish-lc-systems.html. Accessed 7 Jan 2025
29. Antibiotic Testing | Milk Antibiotic Test Kits. https://www.charm.com/products/test-and-kits/antibiotic-tests/. Accessed 7 Jan 2025
30. Food and Beverage Testing. https://sciex.com/applications/food-and-beverage-testing. Accessed 7 Jan 2025
31. Method Development of Ten Antibiotic Compounds Using a Systematic Screening Protocol on an ACQUITY Arc With UV and QDa Detection | Waters. https://www.waters.com/nextgen/in/en/library/application-notes/2021/method-development-of-ten-antibiotic-compounds-using-a-systematic-screening-protocol-on-an-acquity-arc-with-uv-and-qda-detection.html?srsltid=AfmBOoqZB1Bced1BPyVHGqZzLOmnHZ3vtdKuURwAtog49si9Y6jwMewd. Accessed 7 Jan 2025
32. Nanotechnology-Based Biosensors for Biomedical Applications. iopscience.iop.org
33. Khan MQ, Khan J, Alvi MAH, Nawaz H, Fahad M, Umar M (2024) Nanomaterial-based sensors for microbe detection: a review. Discover Nano 19:1–24
34. Next-generation nanophotonic-enabled biosensors for intelligent diagnosis of SARS-CoV-2 variants. Elsevier
35. Abhimanyu, Singh K, Sable H, Sonu S, Kumar V, Singh P, Kaushik A, Thakur P, Chaudhary V (2025) Exploring complex silver sulfide nano-systems as efficient photocatalysts for wastewater remediation and clean energy production: toward sustainable and circular economy. Mater Today. https://doi.org/10.1016/J.MATTOD.2025.09.004
36. Stephen Inbaraj B, Chen BH (2016) Nanomaterial-based sensors for detection of foodborne bacterial pathogens and toxins as well as pork adulteration in meat products. J Food Drug Anal 24:15–28
37. Magro C, Moura T, Dionísio J, Ribeiro PA, Raposo M, Sério S (2022) Nanostructured metal oxide sensors for antibiotic monitoring in mineral and river water. Nano 12:1858
38. Li C, Sun F (2021) Graphene-assisted sensor for rapid detection of antibiotic resistance in Escherichia coli. Front Chem 9:696906
39. Gwyther REA, Côté S, Lee CS, Miao H, Ramakrishnan K, Palma M, Dafydd Jones D (2024) Optimising CNT-FET biosensor design through modelling of biomolecular electrostatic gating and its application to β-lactamase detection. Nature Communications 15:1–10
40. Sansone L, Macchia E, Taddei C, Torsi L, Giordano M (2018) Label-free optical biosensing at femtomolar detection limit. Sens Actuators B Chem 255:1097–1104

41. Herrera-Domínguez M, Morales-Luna G, Mahlknecht J, Cheng Q, Aguilar-Hernández I, Ornelas-Soto N (2023) Optical biosensors and their applications for the detection of water pollutants. Biosensors (Basel) 13:370
42. Nehra M, Kanika, Dilbaghi N, Kumar R, Kumar S (2022) Trends in point-of-care optical biosensors for antibiotics detection in aqueous media. Mater Lett. https://doi.org/10.1016/J.MATLET.2021.131235
43. Chaudhary V, Rustagi S et al (2024 undefined) Perspective—prospect of nano-enabled optical biosensors for antibiotic abuse surveillance as an early prevention tool for antimicrobial resistance. iopscience.iop.org
44. Sun J, Warden AR, Huang J, Wang W, Ding X (2019) Colorimetric and electrochemical detection of Escherichia coli and antibiotic resistance based on a p-Benzoquinone-mediated bioassay. Anal Chem 91:7524–7530
45. Nazemi E, Hassen WM, Frost EH, Dubowski JJ (2017) Monitoring growth and antibiotic susceptibility of Escherichia coli with photoluminescence of GaAs/AlGaAs quantum well microstructures. Biosens Bioelectron 93:234–240
46. Tang Y, Zhen L, Liu J, Wu J (2013) Rapid antibiotic susceptibility testing in a microfluidic pH sensor. Anal Chem 85:2787–2794
47. Nag P, Sadani K, Mukherji S, Mukherji S (2020) Beta-lactam antibiotics induced bacteriolysis on LSPR sensors for assessment of antimicrobial resistance and quantification of antibiotics. Sens Actuators B Chem 311:127945
48. Bi L, Wang X, Cao X, Liu L, Bai C, Zheng Q, Choo J, Chen L (2020) SERS-active Au@Ag core-shell nanorod (Au@AgNR) tags for ultrasensitive bacteria detection and antibiotic-susceptibility testing. Talanta. https://doi.org/10.1016/J.TALANTA.2020.121397
49. Alsaiari NS, Katubi KMM, Alzahrani FM, Siddeeg SM, Tahoon MA (2021) The application of nanomaterials for the electrochemical detection of antibiotics: a review. Micromachines (Basel). https://doi.org/10.3390/MI12030308
50. Kanoun O, Lazarević-Pašti T, Pašti I et al (2021) A review of nanocomposite-modified electrochemical sensors for water quality monitoring. Sensors. https://doi.org/10.3390/S21124131
51. Shi S, Reisberg S, Anquetin G, Noël V, Pham MC, Piro B (2015) General approach for electrochemical detection of persistent pharmaceutical micropollutants: application to acetaminophen. Biosens Bioelectron 72:205–210
52. Sable H, Kumar V, Singh V, Rustagi S, Chaudhary V, Pandit S (2024) Review—nanosystems-enhanced electrochemical biosensors for precision in one health management. J Electrochem Soc 171:037527
53. Hannah S, Dobrea A, Lasserre P, Blair EO, Alcorn D, Hoskisson PA, Corrigan DK (2020) Development of a rapid, antimicrobial susceptibility test for E. coli based on low-cost, screen-printed electrodes. Biosensors 10:153
54. Altobelli E, Mohan R, Mach KE, Sin MLY, Anikst V, Buscarini M, Wong PK, Gau V, Banaei N, Liao JC (2017) Integrated biosensor assay for rapid Uropathogen identification and phenotypic antimicrobial susceptibility testing. Eur Urol Focus 3:293–299
55. Nemr CR, Smith SJ, Liu W, Mepham AH, Mohamadi RM, Labib M, Kelley SO (2019) Nanoparticle-mediated capture and electrochemical detection of methicillin-resistant Staphylococcus aureus. Anal Chem 91:2847–2853
56. Hannah S, Addington E, Alcorn D, Shu W, Hoskisson PA, Corrigan DK (2019) Rapid antibiotic susceptibility testing using low-cost, commercially available screen-printed electrodes. Biosens Bioelectron 145:111696
57. Rueda D, Furukawa R, Fuentes P, Comina G, Rey De Castro NG, Requena D, Gilman RH, Sheen P, Zimic M (2018) A novel inexpensive electrochemical sensor for pyrazinoic acid as a potential tool for the identification of pyrazinamide-resistant Mycobacterium tuberculosis. Int J Mycobacteriol 7:275–281
58. Sitkov NO, Zimina TM, Soloviev AV (2018) Development of impedimetric sensor for E.coli M-17 antibiotic susceptibility testing. In: Proceedings of the 2018 IEEE conference of russian young researchers in electrical and electronic engineering, ElConRus 2018 2018-January, pp 1227–1230

59. Gholipour S, Shamsizadeh Z, Halabowski D, Gwenzi W, Nikaeen M (2024) Combating antibiotic resistance using wastewater surveillance: significance, applications, challenges, and future directions. Sci Total Environ 908:168056
60. Foxman B, Salzman E, Gesierich C, Gardner S, Ammerman M, Eisenberg M, Wigginton K (2024) Wastewater surveillance of antibiotic resistant bacteria for public health action: potential and challenges medRxiv 2024.03.31.24305136
61. Barhoum A, Hamimed S, Slimi H, Othmani A, Abdel-Haleem FM, Bechelany M (2023) Modern designs of electrochemical sensor platforms for environmental analyses: principles, nanofabrication opportunities, and challenges. Trends Environ Anal Chem 38:e00199
62. Talreja RK, Sable H, Chaudhary V, Kadian S, Singh M, Kishore J, Kumar M, Chaudhary V, Khosla A (2024) Challenges in lab-to-clinic translation of 5th/6th generation intelligent nanomaterial-enabled biosensors. ECS Sensors Plus. https://doi.org/10.1149/2754-2726/AD9F7E

Understanding Biosensors, Their Components and Features in the Context of AMR

4

Nikhil Bhalla

4.1 What Is a Biosensor

A biosensor is a device that either detects a biological entity (such as prokaryotic or eukaryotic cells, amino acid- based molecules, or nucleic acid-based molecules) or utilises a biological entity to identify other biological or chemical substances [1]. Biosensors are widely used in fields like healthcare, environmental monitoring, food safety, and biotechnology for their ability to provide accurate, real-time data [2]. They play a crucial role in applications such as disease diagnostics, pollutant detection, and quality control in various industries.

In the context of AMR, biosensors are invaluable tools for early detection of drug-resistant pathogens in clinical, environmental, and agricultural settings. For example, they can identify the presence of resistant strains in patient samples, such as blood or urine [3], within minutes to hours, compared to traditional culture methods that take days. This rapid diagnostic capability supports the implementation of appropriate treatments, reduces the misuse of antibiotics, and helps prevent the spread of resistance [3]. Biosensors are also instrumental in monitoring the levels of antibiotics in environmental samples, such as wastewater and soil, where residual antibiotics can contribute to the emergence of resistance [4]. Additionally, in agriculture, biosensors can detect antibiotic residues in livestock and food products, ensuring compliance with safety regulations and reducing the risk of resistance transfer to humans [5]. The specificity and sensitivity of biosensors enable the detection of resistance mechanisms at the genetic level, such as identifying resistance genes through DNA-based assays [6]. This molecular-level insight helps researchers and healthcare providers understand the mechanisms driving AMR and

N. Bhalla (✉)
Nanotechnology and Integrated Bioengineering Centre (NIBEC), School of Engineering, Ulster University, Belfast, Northern Ireland, UK
e-mail: n.bhalla@ulster.ac.uk

V. Chaudhary, N. Bhalla (eds.), *Biosensors for Tackling Antimicrobial Resistance (AMR)*, https://doi.org/10.1007/978-981-95-9151-0_4

design strategies to counteract them. Furthermore, the portability and cost-effectiveness of many biosensor technologies make them suitable for deployment in resource-limited settings, addressing AMR challenges on a global scale. By facilitating the early detection and monitoring of antimicrobial resistance, biosensors are vital in guiding public health policies, optimising antibiotic stewardship programs, and advancing research into new antimicrobial agents. Their integration into the fight against AMR represents a promising step toward mitigating this growing global health threat.

4.2 Components of a Biosensor

The funcationality of a biosensor is driven by the interplay of five key components: Analyte, Bioreceptor, Transducer, Electronics, and Display.

Analyte The analyte is the substance or molecule of interest that the biosensor is designed to detect. It can be a biological or chemical entity such as: Biomolecules (e.g., glucose, proteins, DNA, or RNA), cells (e.g., bacteria, viruses, or eukaryotic cells) and chemical compounds (e.g., toxins, pollutants, or antibiotics). The analyte is the target of the biosensor's detection process, and its interaction with the bioreceptor initiates the signal generation.

Bioreceptor The bioreceptor is responsible for specifically recognising and interacting with the analyte. It provides the biosensor with its specificity and sensitivity. Examples of bioreceptors include: enzymes which catalyse reactions with specific substrates [7]; cells that detect cellular changes or entire organisms; aptamers which synthetic nucleic acid molecules engineered to bind specific targets [8]; DNA/RNA which can detect complementary nucleic acid sequences and [9]; nanoparticles and nanofilms which may serve as charge sensitive or pH sensitive performing multiple function such as that of a bioreceptor, transducer and signal enhancers [10].

Transducer The transducer converts the interaction between the analyte and bioreceptor into a measurable physical or chemical signal [11, 12]. This signal reflects changes such as elecrtical conducation, light absorbance/emission, heat, pH, or mass change. Some common types of transducers include photodiodes that detect changes in light intensity; Thermistors which measure heat variations; pH Electrodes that monitor pH changes; quartz electrodes that detect mass changes caused by binding events and electrochemical transducers that measures changes electrical activity across the electrode.

Electronics The electronics component processes the raw signal generated by the transducer. It amplifies, converts, and conditions the signal to make it usable and interpretable. Some key process include: analog-to-digital conversion that converts the raw, continuous signal into a digital format for processing and signal conditioning which amplifies and refines the signal to improve clarity and accuracy [13].

Display The display presents the processed signal in a user-friendly format [14–17]. This can be in the format of numerical values which qunatifies the amount of analyte; Graphs which allow visualization of trends or responses (e.g., current vs. potential curves); Visual indicators such as colorimetric or graphical outputs (e.g., 3D models or images).

4.2.1 Processes of Biosensing Components

There are four processes assocaited with the components:

Biorecognition The process begins with the bioreceptor recognising and binding to the analyte. This interaction is usually specific, ensuring the biosensor detects only the target substance.

Signalisation Once the bioreceptor interacts with the analyte, the transducer converts this interaction into a measurable signal. The signal reflects the change caused by the interaction, such as light intensity, heat, pH, or mass alterations.

Quantification The raw signal generated by the transducer is processed for accuracy and usability. The electronics component amplifies, filters, and digitises the signal, ensuring even small changes can be detected and accurately represented.

Output and Interpretation The processed signal is displayed in a readable format. This could be numerical values for precise quantification, graphs to show trends, or visual models for qualitative interpretation. This allows users to analyze the data and make informed decisions.

Figure 4.1 shows compoents and the processes involved in the biosensing.

4.3 Ideal Characteristics of a Biosensor for AMR

Biosensors are indispensable in addressing global health challenges like antimicrobial resistance (AMR) due to their ability to detect specific biomarkers with precision and efficiency. Below are 11 key features that define effective biosensors, also see (Fig. 4.2).

High Sensitivity Sensitivity determines a biosensor's ability to detect low concentrations of a target analyte, such as resistance genes or bacterial toxins. The sensitivity is influenced by the design of self-assembled mono-layers (SAMs) and the transducer properties (e.g., optical or electrochemical). For AMR diagnostics, detecting low levels of bacterial DNA, RNA, or proteins associated with resistance mechanisms without amplification is vital. Techniques such as nanoparticle-enhanced detection and microfluidics are instrumental in improving biosensor sensitivity, enabling detection even at single-molecule levels.

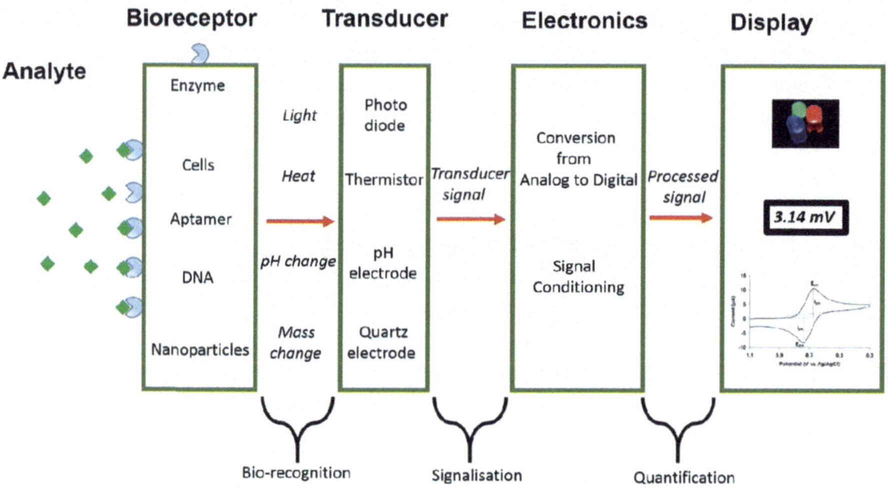

Fig. 4.1 Schematic representation of a biosensor. (Reproduced with permision from [15])

High Selectivity Selectivity refers to a biosensor's capability to detect a target analyte in the presence of homologous molecules and contaminants. For instance, in the context of AMR, biosensors can distinguish bacterial enzymes (e.g., beta-lactamases) that confer resistance from other non-resistance-associated proteins. Achieving high selectivity often involves immobilizing a monolayer of probes, such as aptamers or antibodies, specific to resistance markers on the sensor surface. Developing such selective probes is time-intensive but critical for accurate diagnostics. Advances in nanotechnology, including antifouling coatings and nanomaterial-based surfaces, enable enhanced selectivity by maintaining detection integrity in complex biological samples.

Rapid Response Time The speed at which a biosensor produces results is critical for timely decision-making in AMR management. Ideally, a biosensor should provide results within minutes to guide appropriate antibiotic use. Rapid response is often hindered by post-processing steps like noise reduction or temperature correction. Optimizing signal processing and integrating robust computational methods can minimize delays and enhance real- time applicability.

Multiplexing In cases of AMR, where multiple resistance mechanisms can coexist, the ability to detect multiple biomarkers simultaneously is crucial. Multiplexed biosensors divide the sensing surface into isolated regions, each targeting a specific resistance marker (e.g., different beta-lactamases or efflux pump proteins). This approach enables comprehensive diagnostics and facilitates the identification of co-resistance patterns, improving the precision of treatment strategies.

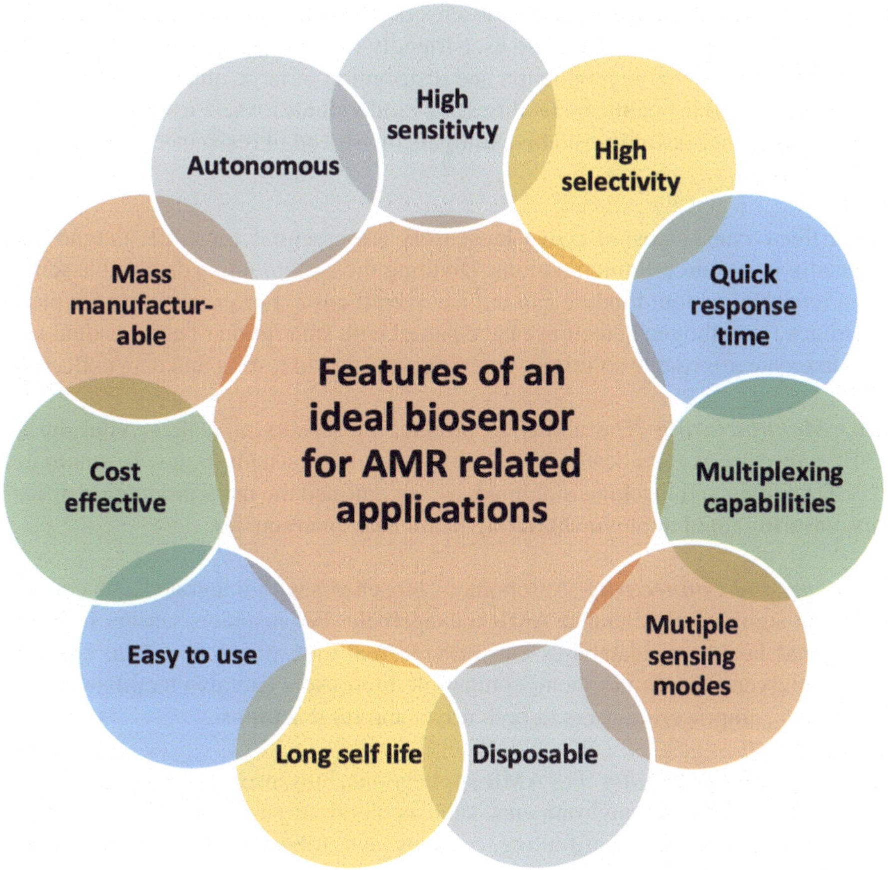

Fig. 4.2 Features of an ideal biosensor required to be developed for effective use in AMR related applications

Multimode Sensing for Validation Multimode sensing increases the reliability of biosensors by using multiple detection mechanisms, such as combining electrochemical and optical techniques. For AMR diagnostics, this could involve cross-validation of resistance biomarkers to ensure robust and accurate results. While multimode sensing may increase sensor complexity and cost, advancements in miniaturization and hybrid platforms are addressing these challenges.

Disposable The infectious nature of resistant pathogens necessitates the use of disposable biosensors to prevent contamination. A modular design, where disposable electrodes are paired with reusable readout modules, is ideal. For AMR applications, materials like paper, plastic, or glass can be used to create cost-effective disposable sensors. Paper-based biosensors, in particular, are gaining attention for their affordability and ease of disposal, making them ideal for use in low-resource settings.

Long Shelf Life and Ease of Use Biosensors for AMR diagnostics should have a shelf life of at least a month and be user-friendly to facilitate widespread adoption. These features enable the production and distribution of large quantities of sensors, which can be used in healthcare facilities or by individuals for self-testing. Simplified designs ensure accessibility and help mitigate the spread of resistance by promoting early detection.

Cost-Effectiveness Cost-effective biosensors are essential for AMR diagnostics, especially in resource-limited regions. Dividing the system into a disposable sensor and a reusable readout module can reduce overall costs. For example, paper-based electrodes for pathogen detection can be paired with smartphone-based readout systems to create affordable solutions, enabling widespread testing and data collection.

Mass Manufacturing The ability to produce biosensors at scale is vital during AMR outbreaks, as early detection is key to containing resistant strains. Technologies like 3D printing and machine molding have streamlined the mass production of sensors, ensuring rapid deployment during healthcare emergencies.

Autonomy and Connectivity Autonomous biosensors with integrated data connectivity can significantly enhance AMR management. For instance, sensors linked to centralized healthcare databases can provide real-time diagnostic data, enabling timely interventions. Smartphone-compatible biosensors can also facilitate remote diagnostics, empowering users in both urban and rural settings.

Robustness and Reliability For AMR applications, biosensors must maintain functionality in challenging environments, such as blood, urine, or other biological fluids. Enhancements like antifouling coatings and robust sensor designs ensure durability and consistent performance, even in complex samples.

By incorporating these features/characteristics, biosensors can play a transformative role in combating AMR, facilitating early detection, personalized treatment, and effective monitoring of resistant infections (Fig. 4.2).

4.4 Where/How Can We Use Biosensor for AMR

In the perspective of AMR biosensors can broadly be utilised in four different fields: (1) clinical diagnostics; (2) food and agriculture monitoring; (3) environmental monitoring and (4) to inform Public health and policies.

4.4.1 Clinical Diagnostics

In healthcare, biosensors play a pivotal role in diagnosing infections and identifying antimicrobial resistance faster than traditional methods like bacterial cultures and susceptibility testing, which are time consuming to perform and at times suffer with false hits. On the other hand biosensors that utilise advanced technologies such as nanoplasmonics, electrochemistry, or fluorescence enable the detection of resistance markers like beta-lactamase enzymes or specific resistance genes directly from patient samples. This rapid detection capability ensures the timely administration of targeted antibiotics, reducing the misuse of broad-spectrum antibiotics and slowing the emergence of resistant strains.

4.4.2 Food and Agriculture Monitoring

AMR also extends to agricultural and food systems where antibiotics are often overused in livestock and aquaculture where biosensors can detect antimicrobial residues in food products and identify resistant pathogens in animals, helping ensure food safety and compliance with regulatory standards. Portable biosensors can also be deployed in real-time during food production or processing to monitor contamination, preventing resistant bacteria from entering the human food chain. Similarly, these devices are invaluable in tracking AMR in aquaculture, where antibiotics are heavily used, leading to environmental contamination.

4.4.3 Environmental Monitoring

The environment is a significant reservoir for AMR, with resistant genes spreading through untreated wastewater and agricultural runoff. Biosensors can detect aAMR-related genetic material or resistant pathogens in water sources, soil, and waste, enabling real-time environmental surveillance. This application is especially critical for identifying contamination hotspots and mitigating the spread of AMR through waterborne or soil-borne pathways.

4.4.4 Public Health and Policy

Biosensors integrated with digital platforms, such as mobile devices or cloud-based systems, provide a scalable solution for AMR surveillance. For instance portable biosensors allow for the collection of real-time data on AMR prevalence in remote or resource-limited settings, where laboratory infrastructure may be insufficient. Such technologies can aid in early outbreak detection, guide treatment protocols, and inform public health policies to combat AMR effectively. By providing actionable insights, biosensors contribute to more efficient decision-making and resource allocation in the global fight against AMR.

4.5 Outlook

This chapter provided a brief background of what a biosensor is and how it can be used for combating AMR. Essentially, biosensors serve as rapid, sensitive, and reliable tools for the detection and monitoring of resistant pathogens and antimicrobial residues. Therefore by develoing innovative components of biosensors such as bioreceptors, transducers, and signal processors, biosensing can bridge the gap between detection of complex biochemical interactions and actionable diagnostic outputs. As the AMR crisis continues to intensify, the development and deployment of biosensors will play an increasingly critical role in mitigating its impact. Advances in nanotechnology, microfluidics, and data integration are pushing the boundaries of biosensor capabilities, enabling portable, low-cost devices that can deliver point-of-care solutions even in resource-limited settings. Furthermore, the in- corporation of artificial intelligence and cloud-based analytics into biosensor platforms holds immense potential for real-time surveillance and predictive modeling, facilitating informed decision-making for healthcare providers and policymakers alike. However, to maximize their impact, several challenges must be addressed, including the standardisation of biosensor performance, scalability of production, and accessibility in low-resource regions. Collaboration among researchers, industry leaders, and governments is essential to ensure biosensors are optimised for practical use and integrated into global strategies for AMR control.

References

1. Bhalla N, Jolly P, Forminsano N, Estrela P (2016) Introduction to biosensors. Essays Biochem 60(1):1–8
2. Chaudhary V, Sable H, Bhadola P (2026) Harnessing complex light-matter interactions for point-of-care nano-optical biosensing. Adv Phys X 11(1):2609776
3. Reynoso EC, Laschi S, Palchetti I, Torres E (2021) Advances in antimicrobial resistance monitoring using sensors and biosensors: a review. Chem 9(8):232
4. Williams A, Aguilar MR, Pattiya Arachchillage KGG et al (2024) Biosensors for public health and environmental monitoring: the case for sustainable biosensing. ACS Sustain Chem Eng 12(28):10296–10312
5. Ribeiro BV, Ferreira LF, Franco DL (2022) Advances in biosensor development for the determination of antibiotics in cow's milk-A review. Talanta Open 6:100145
6. Corbett C-AL, Tardif FJ (2006) Detection of resistance to acetolactate synthase inhibitors in weeds with emphasis on DNA-based techniques: a review. Pest Manage Sci 62(7):584–597
7. Wang X, Zhou J, Wang H (2024) Bioreceptors as the key components for electrochemical biosensing in medicine. Cell Rep Phys Sci 5(2)
8. Liu Q, Chunsheng W, Cai H et al (2014) Cell-based biosensors and their application in biomedicine. Chem Rev 114(12):6423–6461
9. Saadati A, Hassanpour S, de la Guardia M et al (2019) Recent advances on application of peptide nucleic acids as a bioreceptor in biosensors development. TrAC Trends Anal Chem 114:56–68
10. Malekzad H, Zangabad PS, Mirshekari H, Karimi M, Hamblin MR (2017) Noble metal nanoparticles in biosensors: recent studies and applications. Nanotechnol Rev 6(3):301–329

11. Chaudhary V, Sable H, Kumar M, Prakash C, Sonu S (2025) Dynamic landscape of chemiresistive breathomic nanosensors based on fifth-generation chips for complex disease diagnosis and healthcare monitoring. Appl Phys Rev 12(4):041311
12. Sethi RS (1994) Transducer aspects of biosensors. Biosens Bioelectron 9(3):243–264
13. Khiarak MN, Martel S, De Koninck Y, Gosselin B (2019) High-DR CMOS fluorescence biosensor with extended counting ADC and noise cancellation. IEEE Trans Circuits Syst I Regul Pap 66(6):2077–2087
14. Park M (2020) Surface display technology for biosensor applications: a review. Sensors 20(10):2775
15. Bhalla N, Jolly P, Formisano N, Estrela P (2016) Introduction to biosensors. Essays Biochem 60(1):1–8. [Online]. Available: https://doi.org/10.1042/EBC20150001
16. Chaudhary V, Bhadola P (2025) Artificial intelligence-powered nanosensor platforms for non-invasive breathomic diagnostics. Nanotechnol Sci Appl 18:611–641
17. Chaudhary V, Rustagi S, Kaushik A, Bhutani M (2024) Perspective—prospect of nano-enabled optical biosensors for antibiotic abuse surveillance as an early prevention tool for antimicrobial resistance. ECS J Solid State Sci Technol 13(1):017003

Case Studies: Electrical and Electrochemical Biosensors for Antibiotic Abuse Detection

5

Nauman Sadiq, Muafia Akbar, Muhammad Usman, Ghulam Mustafa, and Safeer Ahmed

5.1 Introduction

Antibiotics are a class of very effective antimicrobial substances, and they are used extensively in both human and veterinary medicine to treat a wide range of infectious disorders [1–3]. Types of antibiotics (Fig. 5.1) include tetracyclines, aminoglycoside, cephalosporin, penicillin, macrolides, quinolone, sulfonamides, and trimethoprim [4]. Initially used to treat animal diseases, veterinary antibiotics were widely added to feed for growth promotion and reproduction regulation [5]. Their overuse impacts human health and the environment, with residues persisting as contaminations in water, soil, and foods like meat, milk, fish, poultry, eggs, and honey, posing significant risks [6–8]. Allergy, immunopathological effects, nephropathy, hepatotoxicity, mutagenicity, carcinogenicity, bone marrow toxicity, reproductive problems, and even anaphylactic shock in humans are among the harmful effects that might result from these medications' residues [3, 9, 10].

AMR from antibiotic residues in food is a growing global concern, making some bacterial infections untreatable. To mitigate risks, the European Union banned certain growth promoters. At the same time, the US and Europe set Maximum Residue

N. Sadiq
Department of Chemistry, Quaid-I-Azam University, Islamabad, Pakistan

Department of Chemistry, University of Okara, Okara, Pakistan

M. Akbar · G. Mustafa (✉)
Department of Chemistry, University of Okara, Okara, Pakistan
e-mail: ghulam.mustafa@uo.edu.pk

M. Usman
Department of Electronics, Quaid-I-Azam University, Islamabad, Pakistan

S. Ahmed (✉)
Department of Chemistry, Quaid-I-Azam University, Islamabad, Pakistan
e-mail: safeerad@qau.edu.pk

V. Chaudhary, N. Bhalla (eds.), *Biosensors for Tackling Antimicrobial Resistance (AMR)*, https://doi.org/10.1007/978-981-95-9151-0_5

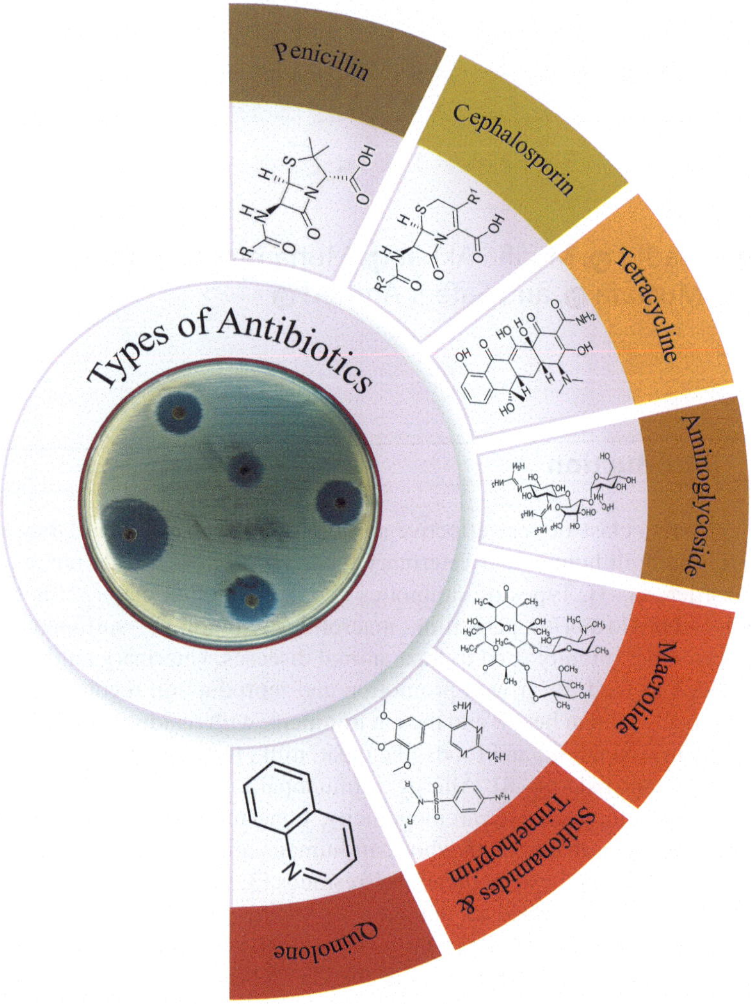

Fig. 5.1 Different types of antibiotics

Limits (MRLs) to ensure safety. Sensitive monitoring techniques are essential to keep antibiotic residues in animal-derived foods below these thresholds [11, 12]. Techniques like GC-MS, LC-MS, and HPLC validate high sensitivity and precision screening results but require expensive instruments, skilled personnel, and lengthy sample preparation [13].

Efforts have focused on developing rapid, affordable, sensitive, and portable biosensors for on-site detection of antibiotic residues, overcoming traditional method limitations. Biosensors enable accurate, real-time monitoring of analytes in food and other fields, effectively detecting antibiotic residues in animal-derived foods. A biosensor integrates a bioreceptor, which interacts specifically with a target analyte, and a transducer, converting the recognition event into a quantifiable signal [14, 15]. Electrochemical biosensors, the most common type, transform biological interactions into measurable signals like voltage or current by detecting changes in electrons or ions in the solution [16–18].

5.2 Electrical Biosensors

Electrical biosensors offer compact, affordable, and low-power solutions for on-site molecular detection and diagnostics by measuring current or voltages [19].

5.2.1 Case Study: Field-Effect Transistor (FET)-Based Biosensor for Antibiotic Abuse Detection

FET-based biosensors detect biological molecules by converting interactions into measurable signals. They comprise a dielectric layer, a semiconductor layer, and three electrodes: the source, drain, and gate [20]. The region between the source and drain is the recognition site, detecting analytes' presence and concentration. Signals can be displayed, processed, or transmitted for analysis [21]. Ion-sensitive and metal-oxide-semiconductor FETs are widely used, differing in gate voltage application and material design, offering high sensitivity and versatility for advanced biosensing applications [22]. A general setup of FET can be seen in Fig. 5.2.

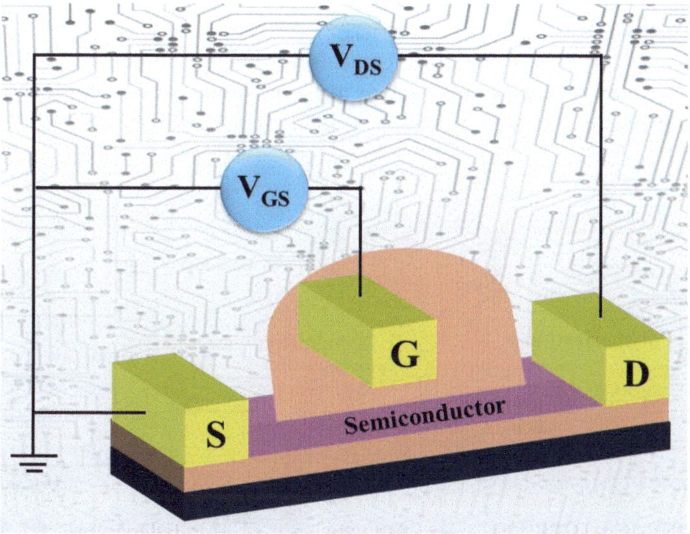

Fig. 5.2 A general setup of FET sensor

The case study of an extended gate field-effect transistor (EGFET) biosensor array for multiple antibiotic detection is discussed [16]. In this study, a dual-recognition strategy was introduced by combining MIPs and aptamers.

5.2.1.1 Methodology

In the dual recognition strategy (Fig. 5.3), MIP provides stability and preconcentration through space-specific binding cavities, and aptamers are highly specific biological probes that bind to antibiotics via unique 3D conformations. To fabricate the EGFET biosensor array, nanosheets of a gold nanoparticle-loaded metal-organic framework are applied to the extended gate electrode. Aptamers were immobilized onto the electrode surface through coordination with Au-S bonds. MIP layer was subsequently employed using controlled surface imprinting via electro-polymerization, ensuring highly specific recognition cavities for target antibiotics. Electro-polymerization cycles, incubation time, and elution processes were optimized for maximum sensitivity and reproducibility.

5.2.1.2 Results

The performance of the EGFET biosensor array was evaluated, and it shows high sensitivity in the femtomolar range. The detection limit for ampicillin, amoxicillin, and kanamycin achieved 4.6 fM, 1.4 fM, and 8.6 fM, respectively. It demonstrated excellent selectivity between target and non-target antibiotics. The sensor's stability was enhanced by providing structural support via the MIP layer and protecting aptamers from degradation. It simultaneously detects all three antibiotics in complex matrices with high recovery rates (80.6–119.2%).

5.2.1.3 Applications

The sensor array effectively identified antibiotics in environmental samples such as tap and river water, food products such as milk and honey, and biological fluids such as artificial urine.

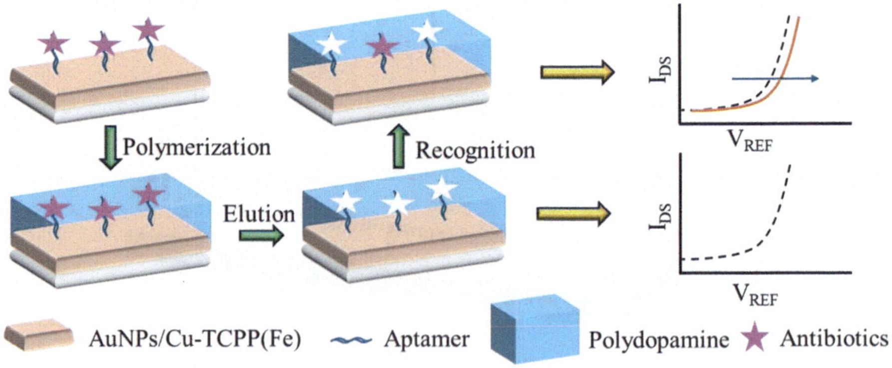

Fig. 5.3 Schematic representation of extended gate electrode functionalized with MIP-aptamer. (Modified from [23])

5.2.2 Case Study: Capacitive Biosensor for Antibiotic Abuse Detection

Capacitive biosensors are label-free devices offering simplicity, low cost, and ultrahigh sensitivity. They consist of a bioreceptor (antibodies and aptamers) and a transducer (carbon, gold, and interdigital electrodes). Biomarker binding alters the dielectric layer's thickness, changing capacitance. Based on the electrical double layer theory [24], these capacitance changes enable biomarker detection, calculated using the following equation.

$$C = \varepsilon\varepsilon_{\circ}\frac{A}{d}$$

ε is the dielectric constant, $\varepsilon_{\circ}$ is vacuum permittivity, A is electrode surface area, and d is the distance between electrodes [25]. An integrated capacitor can be seen in Fig. 5.4.

The case study of a capacitive biosensor for tetracycline antibiotic detection in water samples utilizing an innovative combination of materials and electrical techniques is described [27].

5.2.2.1 Methodology

The capacitive biosensor was developed by an ultrathin-insulating polymer-thiol matrix on a gold electrode for signal transduction. Polytyramine film is formed via the electro-polymerization of tyramine on a gold-coated silicon electrode; this insulating layer provides functional groups for biomolecule attachment. Subsequently, 1-Dodecanethiol fills pinholes in the polymer layer, and polyclonal antibodies specific for tetracycline were attached using 1-ethyl-3-(3-dimethylaminopropyl

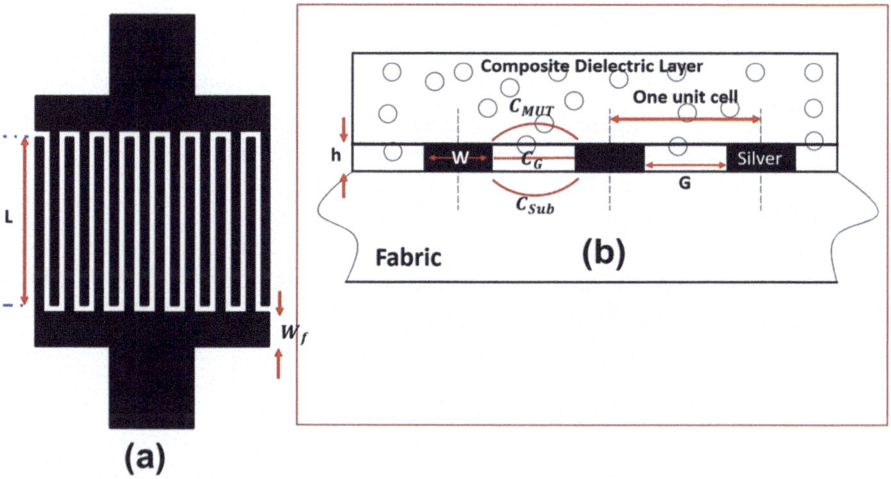

Fig. 5.4 Integrated capacitor (**a**) top and (**b**) cross-sectional view. (Reuse with permission from [26])

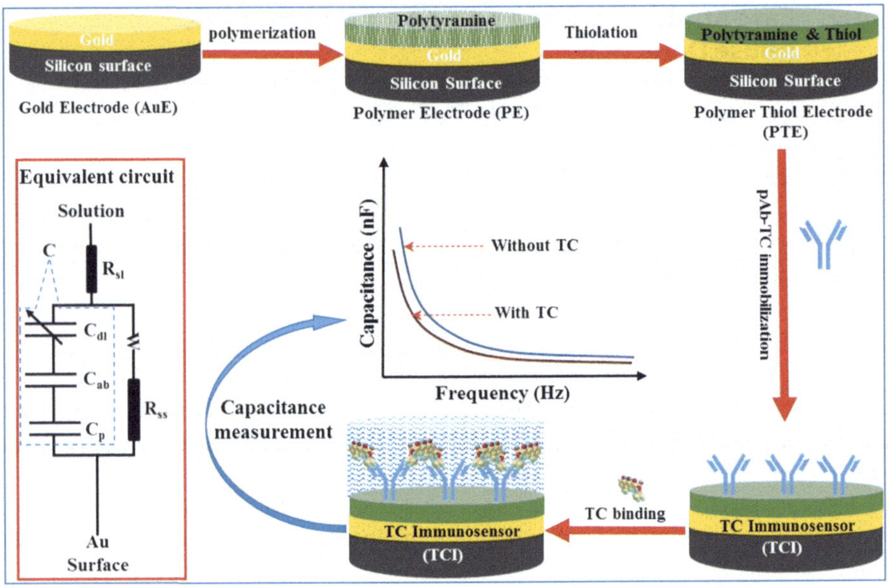

Fig. 5.5 Schematic representation of capacitive biosensor for tetracycline detection with a proposed equivalent circuit. (Reuse with permission from [27])

carbodiimide/N-hydroxysuccinimide coupling chemistry. Furthermore, the surface morphology of the thin surface was confirmed by atomic force microscopy and insulating behavior was evaluated by cyclic voltammetry and capacitive response (Fig. 5.5).

5.2.2.2 Results

The fabricated capacitive biosensor showed a lower limit of detection of 0.01 μg/L for tetracycline and a linear range of 1–200 μg/L. The sensor exhibited high selectivity in the presence of similar (doxycycline) and dissimilar (sulphanilamide) antibiotics. The biosensor performance remained unchanged over four weeks when stored at 4 °C and was reproducible with less than 5% variability.

5.2.2.3 Applications

The biosensor was tested with water samples (tap and bottled) spiked with a known concentration of tetracycline. It exhibited a recovery rate of 96% to 102%, which validated its practical applicability.

5.3 Electrochemical Biosensors

Electrochemical biosensors combine biological recognition elements with transducers for sensitive, specific analyte detection and diagnostics [28, 29].

5.3.1 Case Study: Amperometric Biosensor for Antibiotic Abuse Detection

Amperometric biosensors (Fig. 5.6) measure current from redox reactions at an electrode surface under an applied potential. Electron mediators or nanomaterials enhance detection with the current analyte concentration relationship governed by the Cottrell equation [30].

$$i = \frac{nFAC_{\circ}\sqrt{d}}{\sqrt{\pi t}}$$

A case study of amperometric biosensors for β-lactam antibiotics, such as penicillin G detection in real samples (Milk, Serum, and Urine), which cause or contribute to bacterial resistance [32]. Schematic representation for the detection of penicillin G antibiotic in Fig. 5.7.

5.3.1.1 Methodology

An amperometric biosensor was designed using a polymeric membrane coated with bovine serum albumin conjugated with penicillin G for antibody binding. A transducer of amperometric hydrogen peroxide electrode and avidin-biotin-peroxidase coupling was employed for signal amplification and specificity. Horseradish peroxidase acts as the enzyme maker, producing a measurable amperometric signal upon reaction with hydrogen peroxide. Real samples were spiked with known concentrations of penicillin G to evaluate the sensors' accuracy and recovery rates.

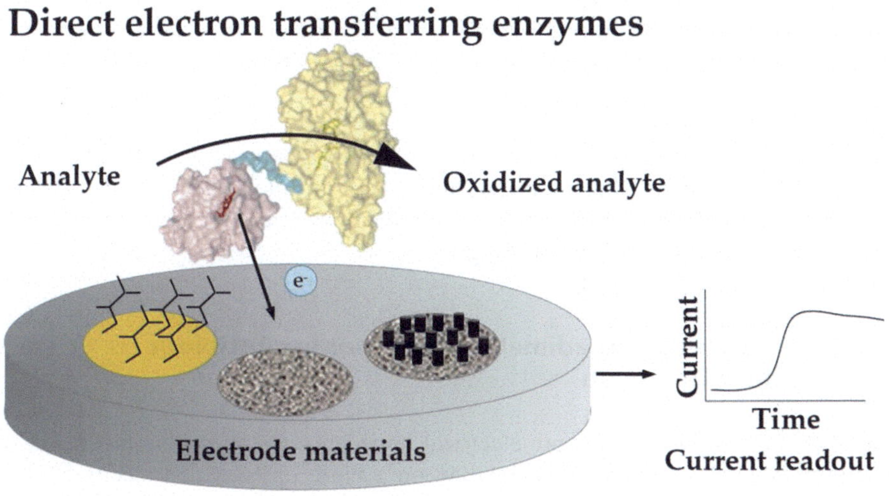

Fig. 5.6 The design of amperometric biosensors [31]

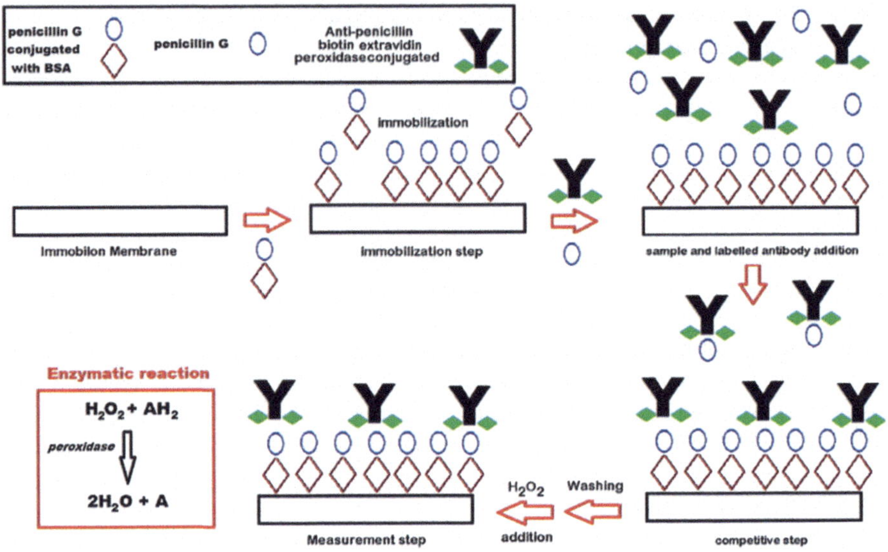

Fig. 5.7 Schematic representation for the detection of penicillin G antibiotic. (Reuse with permission from [32])

5.3.1.2 Results

The developed biosensor showed a lower detection limit of 1.5×10^{-11} M for penicillin G with a linear range of 10^{-11} to 10^{-4} M. It showed excellent selectivity for penicillin G with minimal interference from non-β-lactam antibiotics and other substances. The biosensor's reliability was demonstrated by recovery tests in spiked samples, yielding results between 98.6% and 100.7%. The membrane's regenerating and reusability makes the biosensor stable and reusable.

5.3.1.3 Applications

The amperometric biosensor was applied to test milk samples for penicillin G detection in commercial and infected cow milk. Antibiotic levels were measured in human serum and urine, which are undergoing treatment, and assessed in water resources for environmental monitoring.

5.3.2 Case Study: Impedimetric Biosensor for Antibiotic Abuse Detection

Impedimetric biosensors measure electrical impedance changes from biochemical interactions, such as biomolecule binding on a bioreceptor-coated electrode [33, 34]. Faradic biosensors use redox probes to detect binding through electrochemical activity, while non-faradic electrochemical impedance spectroscopy (EIS) measures dielectric changes at the electrode-electrolyte interface without redox molecules. Non-faradic EIS offers high sensitivity, selectivity, and detection of minimal analyte

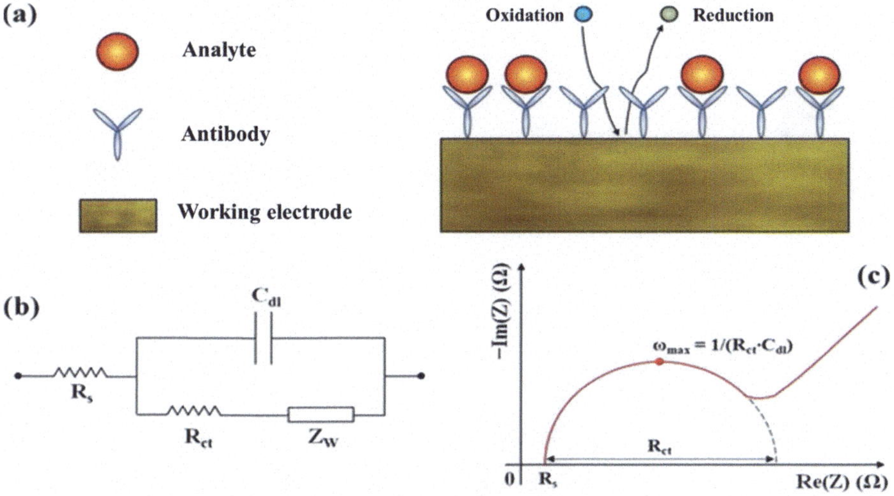

Fig. 5.8 (**a**) Bioreceptor immobilized on the working electrode (**b**) biosensor's equivalent circuit (**c**) Nyquist plot of the circuit. (Modified from [37])

variations [35]. The method involves applying sinusoidal potentials or currents and analyzing the resulting frequency response [36]. A bioreceptor immobilized on the working electrode can be seen in Fig. 5.8.

$$Z(\omega t) = \frac{E(\omega t)}{I(\omega t)}$$

This is a case study of an amperometric biosensor for tobramycin, an aminoglycoside antibiotic detection based on protein-directed carbon nanospheres embedded with SnOx and TiO_2 nanocrystals. This biosensor employs aptamer-based recognition for sensitive and selective detection of tobramycin in aqueous and biological samples.

5.3.2.1 Methodology

A bovine serum albumin template was used to prepare SnOx@TiO_2 nanocomposites. The bovine serum albumin was calcined at temperatures ranging from 300 °C to 900 °C, producing mesoporous carbon nanospheres embedded with SnOx and TiO_2 nanocrystals. The SnOx@TiO_2@mC900 demonstrated the best electrochemical activity for sensor fabrication. Subsequently, a gold electrode was modified with SnOx@TiO_2@mC900 composite. Tobramycin-specific aptamers were immobilized onto the nanocomposite surface, forming the sensitive recognition layer. Aptamer to target binding was monitored through electrochemical impedance spectroscopy, detecting changes in charge transfer resistance upon tobramycin interaction (Fig. 5.9).

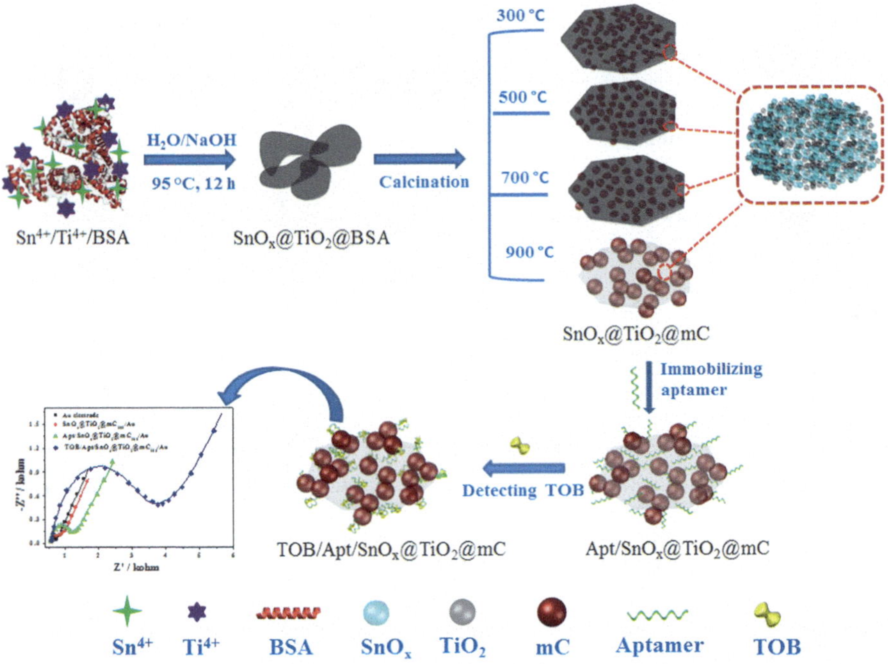

Fig. 5.9 Schematic representation of the preparation of bovine serum albumin-directed SnOx@ TiO_2@mC composite and detection of tobramycin. (Reuse with permission of [38])

5.3.2.2 Results

The tobramycin detection was tested in aqueous solutions, human serum, and urine samples spiked with known tobramycin concentrations. The biosensor achieved a limit of detection of 6.7 pg/mL with a linear dynamic detection range of 0.01 ng/mL to 5 ng/mL. High specificity was observed for tobramycin with negligible interference from other antibiotics such as kanamycin and streptomycin and biomolecules like glucose and amino acids. The sensor retained 90% of its initial sensitivity after 15 days of storage at 4 °C exhibited its stability and reproducible with a 4.3% relative standard deviation.

5.3.2.3 Applications

The fabricated impedimetric biosensor was employed in human serum and urine samples, and tobramycin recovery ranged from 90.2% to 108.5%, showcasing high accuracy and potential for clinical applications.

5.3.3 Case Study: Potentiometric Biosensor for Antibiotic Abuse Detection

A potentiometric biosensor (Fig. 5.10) integrates a biological sensing element with an electrochemical potential transducer [39]. It relies on biochemical reactions,

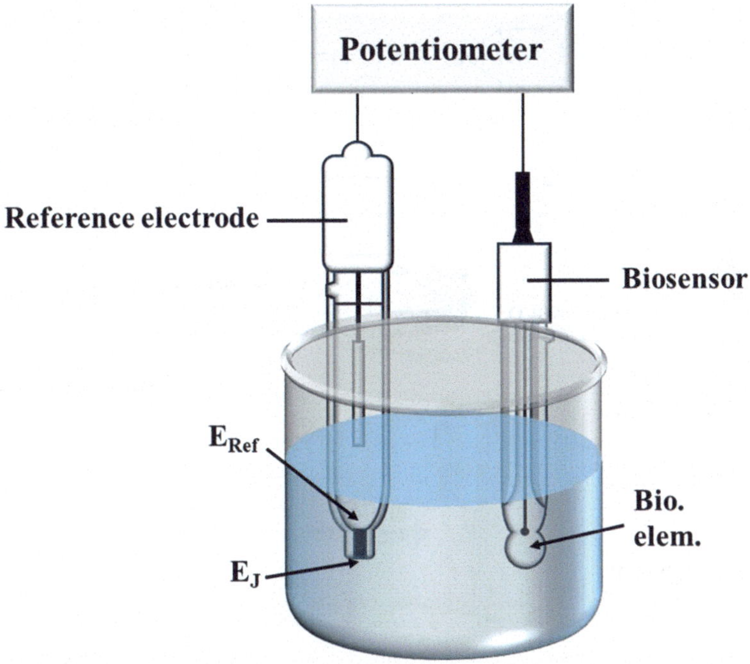

Fig. 5.10 Diagram of potentiometric biosensor. (Modified from [41])

often enzyme-catalyzed, to produce ions near an ion-sensitive electrode. An electrochemical cell with ion-selective and reference electrodes measures potential differences without current flow. These compact, rapid, cost-effective sensors resist interferences like color and require minimal sample volume [40]. Using the Nernst equation, their analytical signal determines the concentration of specific solution components.

$$E = E^{\circ} + \frac{RT}{nF}\ln\left[a_i\right]$$

E is the potential, R is the gas coefficient (8.314 J/K), F is the Faraday constant (96,500 C/mol), n is the number of electrons, and a_i is the ion activity. E° is the standard potential.

A case study of potentiometric biosensor based on aptamer for the sensitive and selective detection of chloramphenicol, a broad-spectrum antibiotic with adverse effects such as aplastic anemia and genotoxicity in humans (Fig. 5.11) [42].

5.3.3.1 Methodology

The potentiometric biosensor was fabricated by a screen-printed graphite electrode modified with mesoporous silica functionalized by 1,4-diazabicyclo[2.2.2]octane that enhances the surface area. It is modified with dendritic gold nanostructures via electrochemical deposition to improve conductivity and immobilize thiolated

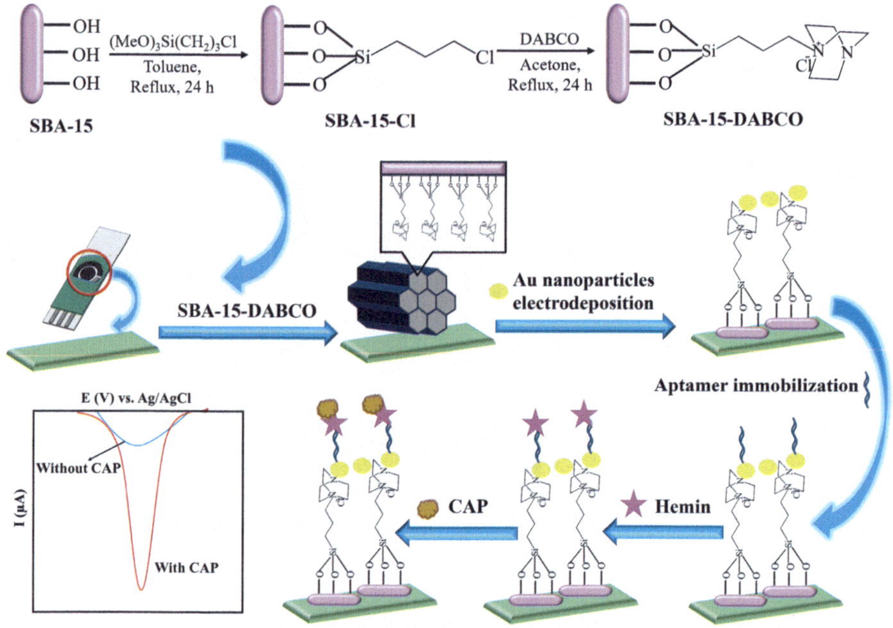

Fig. 5.11 Scheme of developing a potentiometric biosensor for detecting chloramphenicol. (Modified from [42])

chloramphenicol binding aptamer via Au-S bonds an electrochemical indicator, hemin, interacted with the aptamer's guanine bases. The aptamer folds and stabilizes, enhancing the interaction with hemin when chloramphenicol binds and generates an amplified DPV signal proportional to chloramphenicol concentration.

5.3.3.2 Results

The designed sensor exhibited linear detection ranges of 0.03–0.15 μM and 0.15–7.0 μM, with a detection limit of 4.0 nM. High selectivity was confirmed through negligible cross-reactivity with other antibiotics, such as amoxicillin and florfenicol. The sensor showed consistent responses with a relative standard deviation of 1.2%.

5.3.3.3 Applications

Spike and recovery experiments evaluated the sensor performance in human serum samples. The recovery rates were 90–93%, demonstrating its feasibility for real-world applications.

5.4 Comparison of Case Studies

The case studies compare electrical and electrochemical biosensors for antibiotic detection. Technologically, electrical biosensors enhance real-time signals and improve robustness and multiplexing. Electrochemical biosensors utilize redox reactions or impedance changes for high specificity but often require sophisticated material modifications. Electrical biosensors achieve femtomolar sensitivity and excel in multiplex detection, while electrochemical offer comparable sensitivity, broader detection ranges, and practical usability in complex samples. Both techniques exhibit high selectivity. Stability remains an issue, with aptamer degradation or electrode fouling affecting reusability. Fabrication costs and reproducibility across sensors also limit scalability. Despite differences, both platforms provide cost-effective, scalable alternatives to conventional antibiotic detection methods.

5.5 Conclusions

The overuse of antibiotics has escalated AMR into a global health crisis, emphasizing the need for rapid, accurate detection methods across environmental, clinical, and food matrices. Electrical and electrochemical biosensors have emerged as powerful tools for addressing this challenge, offering sensitive, real-time, cost-effective solutions and bridging the gap between laboratory research and practical use. By integrating advanced materials such as nanostructures, MIPs, and aptamers, these biosensors provide scalable and portable solutions for healthcare, food safety, and environmental monitoring. Future improvements should address long-term stability, reproducibility, and cost. Enhancing material robustness, optimizing electrode interfaces, and developing more efficient regeneration methods will be crucial for extending biosensor lifespans. Future opportunities lie in expanding multiplex detection capabilities to monitor diverse targets simultaneously, which are essential for complex real-world samples. Miniaturization and integration of biosensors with digital technologies, such as IoT-enabled systems and AI-based data processing, could revolutionize point-of-care diagnostics and environment surveillance. These advancements will pave the way for next-generation biosensor platforms.

References

1. Sharma A, Istamboulie G, Hayat A, Catanante G, Bhand S, Marty JL (2017) Disposable and portable aptamer functionalized impedimetric sensor for detection of kanamycin residue in milk sample. Sensors Actuators B Chem 245:507–515
2. Pal A, Sable H, Uniyal A, Chaudhary V (2025) Green Nano-semiconductors and nanometals to avert complex phenomena of antimicrobial resistance (AMR). Current Opinion in Biomed Eng 36:100626
3. Singh V, Sable H, Ghalley M, Tenzin K. Environmental toxicology, fate and risk assessment of emerging contaminants. Occurrence, distribution and toxic effects of emerging contaminantsx: CRC Press; 2024. 134–167
4. Gaudin V (2017) Advances in biosensor development for the screening of antibiotic residues in food products of animal origin a comprehensive review. Biosens Bioelectron 90:363–377
5. Ngangom BL, Tamunjoh SSA, Boyom FF (2019) Antibiotic residues in food animals: public health concern. Acta Ecol Sin 39(5):411–415
6. Kolpin DW, Furlong ET, Meyer MT, Thurman EM, Zaugg SD, Barber LB et al (2002) Pharmaceuticals, hormones, and other organic wastewater contaminants in US streams, 1999–2000: A national reconnaissance. Environ Sci Technol 36(6):1202–1211

7. Sable H, Kumar V, Singh V, Rustagi S, Chahal S, Chaudhary V (2024) Strategically engineering advanced nanomaterials for heavy-metal remediation from wastewater. Coord Chem Rev 518:216079
8. Sable H, Singh V, Kumar V, Roy A, Pandit S, Kaur K et al (2024) Toxicological and bioremediation profiling of nonessential heavy metals (mercury, chromium, cadmium, aluminium) and their impact on human health: a review. Toxicologie Analytique et Clinique 36(3):205–234
9. Bacanlı M, Başaran N (2019) Importance of antibiotic residues in animal food. Food Chem Toxicol 125:462–466
10. Chaudhary V, Sable H, Kumar M, Prakash C, Sonu S (2025) Dynamic landscape of chemiresistive breathomic nanosensors based on fifth-generation chips for complex disease diagnosis and healthcare monitoring. Applied Phys Rev 12(4)
11. Leibovici L, Paul M, Garner P, Sinclair DJ, Afshari A, Pace NL et al (2016) Addressing resistance to antibiotics in systematic reviews of antibiotic interventions. J Antimicrob Chemother 71(9):2367–2369
12. Directive EC (2002) 657/EC of 12 August, 1990 On implementing Council Directive 96/23/EC concerning the performance of analytical methods and the interpretation of results. Off J Eur Communities L221
13. Chiesa LM, Nobile M, Panseri S, Arioli F (2017) Antibiotic use in heavy pigs: comparison between urine and muscle samples from food chain animals analysed by HPLC-MS/MS. Food Chem 235:111–118
14. Hlabangana L, Memeza S (2018) Ion-pair isocratic simultaneous determination of broad spectrum antibiotics in environmental samples by HPLC with UV detection. Environ Nanotechnol Monitor Manag 10:104–111
15. Thévenot DR, Toth K, Durst RA, Wilson GS (2001) Electrochemical biosensors: recommended definitions and classification. Biosens Bioelectron 16(1–2):121–131
16. Tomassetti M, Serone M, Angeloni R, Campanella L, Mazzone E (2015) Amperometric enzyme sensor to check the total antioxidant capacity of several mixed berries. Comparison with two other spectrophotometric and fluorimetric methods. Sensors 15(2):3435–3452
17. Chaudhary V, Lucky L, Sable H, Bhalla N (2025) Interdisciplinary approach to Monkeypox prevention: integrating nanobiosensors, nanovaccines, artificial intelligence, visual arts, and social sciences. Small Struct 6:2400647
18. Sable H, Kumar V, Singh V, Rustagi S, Chaudhary V, Pandit S (2024) Nanosystems-enhanced electrochemical biosensors for precision in one health management. J Electrochem Soc 171(3):037527
19. Choi J, Seong TW, Jeun M, Lee KH (2017) Field-effect biosensors for on-site detection: recent advances and promising targets. Adv Healthc Mater 6(20):1700796
20. Nguyen TT-H, Nguyen CM, Huynh MA, Vu HH, Nguyen T-K, Nguyen N-T (2023) Field effect transistor based wearable biosensors for healthcare monitoring. J Nanobiotechnol 21(1):411
21. Wadhera T, Kakkar D, Wadhwa G, Raj B (2019) Recent advances and progress in development of the field effect transistor biosensor: a review. J Electron Mater 48:7635–7646
22. Sadighbayan D, Hasanzadeh M, Ghafar-Zadeh E (2020) Biosensing based on field-effect transistors (FET): recent progress and challenges. TrAC Trends Anal Chem 133:116067
23. Tao T, Wei X, Ye Z, Zong B, Li Q, Mao S (2024) Dual recognition strategy-based transistor sensor Array for ultrasensitive and multi-target detection of antibiotics. Adv Funct Mater 35:2413485
24. Tsouti V, Boutopoulos C, Zergioti I, Chatzandroulis S (2011) Capacitive microsystems for biological sensing. Biosens Bioelectron 27(1):1–11
25. Ahn J, Lee TH, Li T, Heo K, Hong S, Ko J et al (2011) Electrical immunosensor based on a submicron-gap interdigitated electrode and gold enhancement. Biosens Bioelectron 26(12):4690–4696
26. Truong T, Kim J-S, Yeun E, Kim J (2022) Wearable capacitive pressure sensor using interdigitated capacitor printed on fabric. Fash Text 9(1):46

27. Prusty AK, Bhand S (2020) A capacitive immunosensor for tetracycline estimation using antibody modified polytyramine-alkanethiol ultra-thin film on gold. J Electroanal Chem 863:114055
28. Wu J, Liu H, Chen W, Ma B, Ju H (2023) Device integration of electrochemical biosensors. Nat Rev Bioeng 1(5):346–360
29. Chaudhary V, Bhadola P (2025) Artificial intelligence-powered nanosensor platforms for non-invasive breathomic diagnostics. Nanotechnol Sci Appl Volume 18:611–641
30. Apetrei C, Ghasemi-Varnamkhasti M (2013) Biosensors in food PDO authentication. In: Comprehensive analytical chemistry, vol 60. Elsevier, pp 279–297
31. Schachinger F, Chang H, Scheiblbrandner S, Ludwig R (2021) Amperometric biosensors based on direct electron transfer enzymes. Molecules 26(15):4525
32. Merola G, Martini E, Tomassetti M, Campanella L (2015) Simple and suitable immunosensor for β-lactam antibiotics analysis in real matrixes: Milk, serum, urine. J Pharm Biomed Anal 106:186–196
33. Štukovnik Z, Fuchs-Godec R, Bren U (2023) Nanomaterials and their recent applications in impedimetric biosensing. Biosensors 13(10):899
34. Yang L, Guiseppi-Elie A (2008) Impedimetric biosensors for nano-and microfluidics. In: Encyclopedia of microfluidics and nanofluidics, pp 811–823
35. Upasham S, Banga IK, Jagannath B, Paul A, Lin K-C, Muthukumar S et al (2021) Electrochemical impedimetric biosensors, featuring the use of room temperature ionic liquids (RTILs): special focus on non-faradaic sensing. Biosens Bioelectron 177:112940
36. Štukovnik Z, Bren U (2022) Recent developments in electrochemical-impedimetric biosensors for virus detection. Int J Mol Sci 23(24):15922
37. Grossi M, Riccò B (2017) Electrical impedance spectroscopy (EIS) for biological analysis and food characterization: a review. J Sensor Sensor Syst 6(2):303–325
38. Wang M, Hu B, Yang C, Zhang Z, He L, Fang S et al (2018) Electrochemical biosensing based on protein-directed carbon nanospheres embedded with SnOx and TiO2 nanocrystals for sensitive detection of tobramycin. Biosens Bioelectron 99:176–185
39. Yunus S, Jonas AM, Lakard B (2013) Potentiometric biosensors. In: Roberts GCK (ed) Encyclopedia of biophysics. Springer Berlin Heidelberg, Berlin, Heidelberg, pp 1941–1946
40. Wang C, Liu M, Wang Z, Li S, Deng Y, He N (2021) Point-of-care diagnostics for infectious diseases: from methods to devices. Nano Today 37:101092
41. Kubota LT, Da Silva JAF, Sena MM, Alves WA (2022) Tools and trends in bioanalytical chemistry. Springer
42. Bagheri Hashkavayi A, Raoof JB, Azimi R, Ojani R (2016) Label-free and sensitive aptasensor based on dendritic gold nanostructures on functionalized SBA-15 for determination of chloramphenicol. Anal Bioanal Chem 408:2557–2565

Case Studies: Optical Biosensors for Antibiotic Abuse Detection

6

Vatika Soni, Akshay Chawla, Diksha Pathania, Pardeep Singh, and Sonu Sonu

6.1 Introduction

The unnecessary as well as uncontrolled use of antibiotics in veterinary treatment and industries related to food has led to antibiotic resistance, a serious global health concern. Antibiotics are mainly directed to livestock in order to prevent disease, to promote growth and for various therapeutic purposes, resulting in the accumulation of various antibiotic residues in meat, milk, eggs etc. like animal-derived foodstuffs [1, 2]. The presence of these antibiotic residues in the food chain mainly poses serious health risks for example; the generation of different antibiotic-resistant bacteria, treatment failures, increased morbidity as well as mortality rates [3, 4]. To mitigate these associated risks, strict guidelines have been established to monitor as well as control the antibiotic remains in food. Various conventional confirmatory approaches, for example; liquid chromatography-mass spectrometry and electrophoretic methods give high accuracy data but may require extensive sample preparation, skilled staffs, as well as sophisticated instrumentation [4, 5]. Biosensors are advanced analytical tools that associate biological recognition elements along with physical and chemical transducers in order to detect and measure various specific analytes with high accuracy. These devices are instrumental in medical diagnostics, monitoring environment, food safety, and biotechnology like extensive range of fields as shown in Fig. 6.1a [6]. A biosensor's core functionality lies in its capacity to convert or translate a biological interaction into a measurable signal, making it a significant component in addressing contemporary analytical as well as diagnostic challenges

V. Soni · A. Chawla · P. Singh · S. Sonu (✉)
School of Advanced Chemical Sciences, Shoolini University, Solan, HP, India

D. Pathania
Dairy Technology Division, National Dairy Research Institute (ICAR),
Karnal, Haryana, India

V. Chaudhary, N. Bhalla (eds.), *Biosensors for Tackling Antimicrobial Resistance (AMR)*, https://doi.org/10.1007/978-981-95-9151-0_6

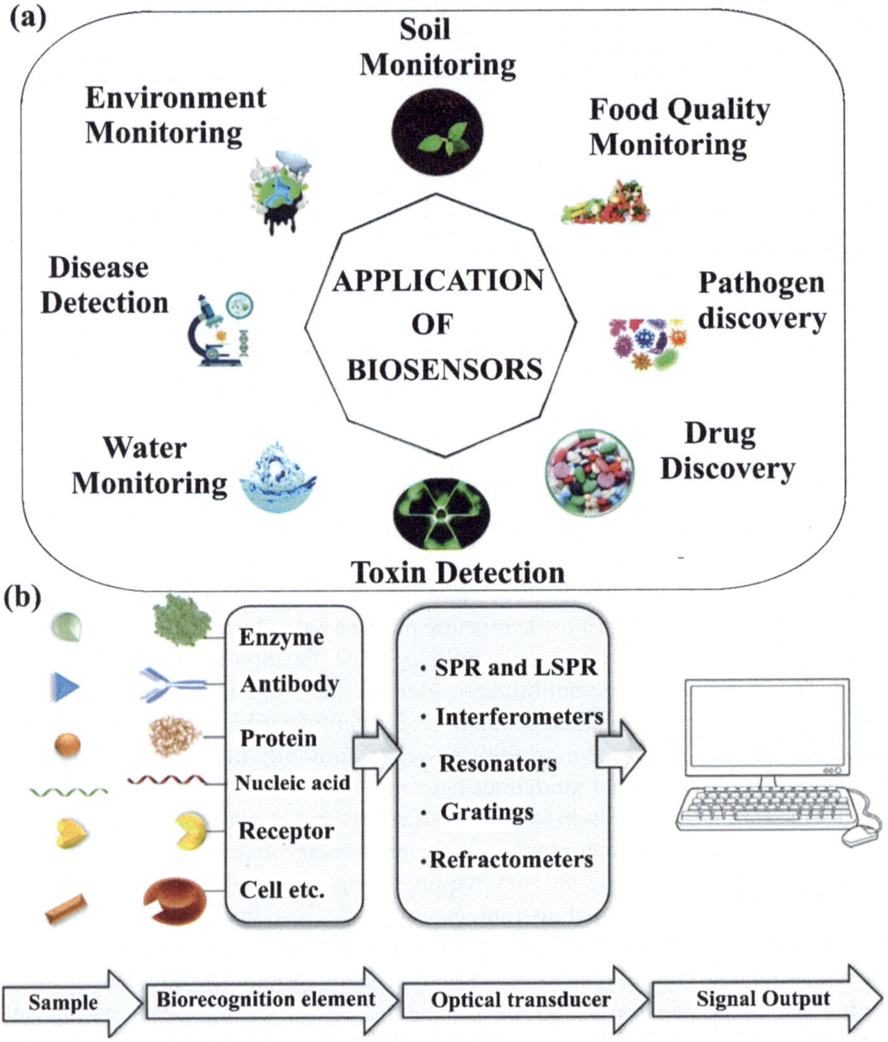

Fig. 6.1 (**a**) Different applications of biosensors. (Adapted with permission from Ref. [6]; Licence No. CC BY 4.0) (**b**) Demonstrated scheme of an optical biosensor along with its fundamental components, (Reprinted with permission from Ref. [28]; Licence No. CC BY)

[7, 8]. Among different types of biosensors, optical biosensors stand out owing to their high sensitivity, specificity, as well as efficacy to deliver real-time results.

Optical biosensors, offer a promising substitute owing to their high sensitivity, rapid detection, as well as easy operational efficiency. These biosensors use light-based detection system to deliver real-time monitoring of antibiotic remains, making them an effective tool for wide-scale applications in biotechnology, slaughterhouses, environmental and food safety monitoring, farms [9, 10]. Optical biosensors use alterations in fluorescence, absorbance, refractive index, or light scattering like optical characteristics during the interaction of an analyte with a bioreceptor. These sensors mainly provide non-invasive as well as highly accurate methods of detection, allowing the discovery of target molecules even at very lower concentrations. Their adaptability has made them efficient in detecting pathogens, measuring environmental contaminants, as well as monitoring therapeutic drug levels like applications [11]. The rising interest in optical biosensors is driven by developments in nanotechnology, material science, as well as data processing techniques. The integration of nanomaterials such as quantum dots, nanoparticles, and nanowires has significantly enhanced the performance of optical biosensors by enhancing their sensitivity as well as increasing their detection range. Moreover, the development of portable as well as user-friendly optical biosensors has extended their accessibility, making them appropriate for point-of-care diagnostics as well as on-site environmental assessments [12]. Optical biosensors can be mainly classified into various groups on the basis of their transduction mechanism, including fluorescence-based biosensors, surface plasmon resonance biosensors, fiber-optic biosensors, as well as nanomaterial-enhanced optical biosensors. Each type provides different advantages in terms of detection real time monitoring, sensitivity as well as selectivity [13, 14].

Fluorescence biosensors mainly depend on the emission of different fluorescent signals when interact with the target analyte. They use quantum dots, fluorescent dyes, and genetically modified fluorescent proteins to spot biomolecules with higher specificity. Their efficiency to offer rapid as well as extremely sensitive detection makes them broadly used in different fields like; biomedical diagnostics, monitoring of environment, food safety assessments etc. mainly for the detection of pathogens, toxins, as well as antibiotic residues [15–17]. Surface Plasmon Resonance biosensor's function significantly based on the principle of surface plasmon resonance, where alteration in the value of refractive index at the surface of sensor are measured in real time [18]. This label-free detection route allows the monitoring of biomolecular interactions that make it a significant tool in drug discovery, immunochemical assay, as well as antibiotic residue discovery. The sensitivity of surface plasmon resonance biosensors allows for the quantification of even minute antibiotics amount in the food [19–21]. Another, fiber optic biosensors use optical fibers to transmit as well as to collect the light, allowing remote/in situ discovery of selected analytes [22]. They are highly advantageous for their flexibility, miniaturization, and ability to operate in harsh environments. They are mainly employed in environmental monitoring, food safety, as well as medical diagnostics owing to their sensitivity and fast response time. In the detection of antibiotics, fiber optic biosensors significantly improve the real-time examination of residues in meat as well dairy foodstuffs [23]. The integration of different nanomaterials, for example; Au nanoparticles, carbon nanotubes, quantum dots, etc. has significantly enhanced the efficiency of optical biosensors. These nanomaterial-improved biosensors provide higher sensitivity, lower detection limits, as well as higher stability, making them efficient for detecting the residues of antibiotic in food as well as biological samples [24]. The utilization of nanostructured surfaces intensifies the signal transduction, allowing precise as well as ultrasensitive analysis of trace antibiotic contamination

[25]. These optical biosensors play a significant role in the detection of antibiotic residue, providing rapid, precise, as well as cost-effective techniques to address the associated challenges with misuse of antibiotics and their influence on the public health. This book chapter mainly explores the efficacy of optical biosensors for the detection of antibiotic abuse, highlighting their principles, advantages, and their real-world applications. By offering a cost-effective solution, optical biosensors show a significant role in confirming the safety of food and reducing the rising risk of antibiotic resistance.

6.2 Fundamentals of Optical Biosensors

Optical biosensors are analytical devices that use optical principles to identify biological interactions with high sensitivity as well as specificity in real time. They integrate a biological recognition element along with a transducer that significantly converts a biological interaction into assessable optical signals. Their capability to provide rapid, precise, and label-free detection makes them extensively applicable in various fields [26, 27]. The main components as well as principles that define the optical biosensors are highlighted below (Fig. 6.1b) [28].

6.2.1 Biological Recognition Element

The biological recognition element, often called as the bioreceptor, as it is mainly responsible for interacting selectively with the target analyte to form a measurable complex. The choice of bioreceptor regulates the specificity as well as sensitivity of the optical biosensor [29]. Common biological recognition elements include: (a) Antibodies are mainly used in immunochemical assay owing to their specificity to detect antigen. Antibody-based optical biosensors are mainly utilised to recognize different pathogens, toxins, and residues of antibiotics. (b) Enzymatic biosensors mainly catalyse specific reactions that generate noticeable optical changes like fluorescence/colorimetric shifts. These biosensors are very specific and effective to detect small molecules, including antibiotics as well as metabolic byproducts [30]. (c) Single-stranded deoxy-ribose or ribose nucleic acids probes provide hybridization-based sensing to detect specific genomic sequences. This mechanism is significant to detect antibiotic resistance genes in different bacterial strains. (d) Aptamers are synthetic oligonucleotides that show high affinity as well as specificity for different target antibiotics and proteins molecules. Aptamer-based optical biosensors are an evolving class owing to their stability and ease of alteration [31]. (e) Whole-cell biosensors use living cells/microorganisms as recognition elements to detect substances through their cellular responses. These biosensors are highly valuable to monitor environment as well as toxicity assessments [32].

6.2.2 Optical Transduction Mechanism

The optical transducer significantly converts the biological interaction into an assessable optical signal. The selection of the transduction mechanism effects the sensitivity, specificity, and detection limit efficiency of biosensors [33]. The commonly used optical transduction mechanisms include: (a) Absorbance: It measures variation in the light absorption due to the presence of the analyte or its products and is widely utilized in biosensors where the binding event leads to a colour change that is visible to eyes. (b) Fluorescence-based biosensors detect the released light due to excitation from fluorophores. This method offers high sensitivity and is used to spot low-concentration antibiotic residues as well as biomolecules [34]. Surface Plasmon Resonance biosensors monitor variation in the refractive index value near a metal surface. This resonance technique allows label-free detection as well as monitoring (real-time) of binding events, making this technique apt for drug discovery as well as to detect antibiotics [35]. (c) Interferometry technique exploits different phase shifts/interference patterns in light waves mainly caused by analyte-sensor binding. These biosensors are extremely sensitive and mainly utilized to detect various molecular interactions [36]. (d) Raman Spectroscopy use inelastic light scattering to offer specific molecular fingerprints of analyte. Raman-based biosensors are mainly utilized for high-specificity chemical as well as molecular identification [37].

6.2.3 Sensing Mechanisms

Optical biosensors offer various sensing strategies to detect different analytes having their own advantages and applications. The sensing mechanisms include: (a) Label-Free Detection approach that depends on the intrinsic optical characteristics of the analyte, for example; variation in refractive index value, scattering of light, or absorbance, eliminating the requirement for labels [29]. They are widely utilized in real-time monitoring of biomolecular interactions. (b) In Label-Based Detection various labels like fluoro/chromophores, or nanoparticles are utilized to intensify the detection signal. Both fluorescent as well as colorimetric biosensors primarily depend on label-based detection mechanism to achieve high sensitivity to detect antibiotics and toxins [38]. (c) Localized Plasmon Resonance biosensors use the exceptional optical characteristics of Au and Ag metallic nanoparticles, to improve the sensitivity and offer colorimetric responses [39]. They are highly efficient to detect low-concentration analytes in food as well as environmental applications.

The fundamentals of optical biosensors mainly revolve around the combination of biological recognition particles along with optical transduction mechanisms to attain highly sensitive as well as specific analyte discovery. These abovementioned biosensors have developed the field of analytical sensing by providing real-time, fast, as well as non-invasive detection abilities [40]. Despite various associated challenges including stability, environmental factors, as well as formation complexity, the ongoing improvements in nanotechnology along with bioengineering continue to boost the efficiency of optical biosensors. Their application in detecting antibiotic residue, medical diagnostics, as well as monitoring of environment highlights their essential role in recent analytical science.

6.3 Application of Optical Biosensor for Antibiotic Detection

Optical biosensors are very important for medical diagnosis and food safety because of how sensitive and easy they are to use [29]. This section demonstrates their versatility across numerous industries by discussing their main uses and the significant advancements that have taken place in the last decade. The pharmaceutical industry, healthcare, quality control in food and drink, monitoring of industrial processes, veterinary and agricultural operations, diagnosis and treatment of illness, biotechnology, defence and military operations, and environmental monitoring are among the most prevalent applications (Fig. 6.2) [41, 42]. Optical biosensors' application in pharmaceutical research, environmental monitoring, clinical diagnostics, and food processing has grown in popularity during the last several years. They are ideal for environmental and industrial uses, especially for detecting antibiotic residue, owing to their resilience, reliability, and ability to decrease outside impact. In contrast to detection approaches based on molecular labelling, optical biosensors do not need complex sample pre-treatment that might alter target molecules, specialized equipment, or specific data processing. This benefit expands their utilisation and potential applications in the real world.

(a) **Antibiotics detection in Food**

The miniaturization of optical biosensors makes them ideal for application in chip-based systems. For compact and adaptable uses, microfluidics might pave the way for lab-on-a-chip devices [43]. The advantages of optical transducers over thermal or piezoelectric detection systems are their sensitivity, stability, resistance to interference from outside sources, and low noise output (Fig. 6.3) [44]. Optical biosensors are able to improve clinical diagnostics, drug development, food quality control, and environmental monitoring thanks to these characteristics, which enable them to efficiently evaluate biological systems. Additionally, these sensors outperform label-based sensors due to the fact that they do away with costly pretreatment processes and block interference from target molecules [45, 46]. The aptamer modification procedures for optical aptasensors are specified by the detection measurement method.

Fluorescent Biosensor

Ensuring the safety and quality of food relies heavily on biosensors, especially those that can detect infections and toxins [47]. Recent advances in optical biosensors have allowed for more precise detection of bacteria, antibiotics, and pesticides, as well as better quality control in food processing [48]. The use of optical biosensors in the inspection of food and drink for contaminants and potential toxicity is

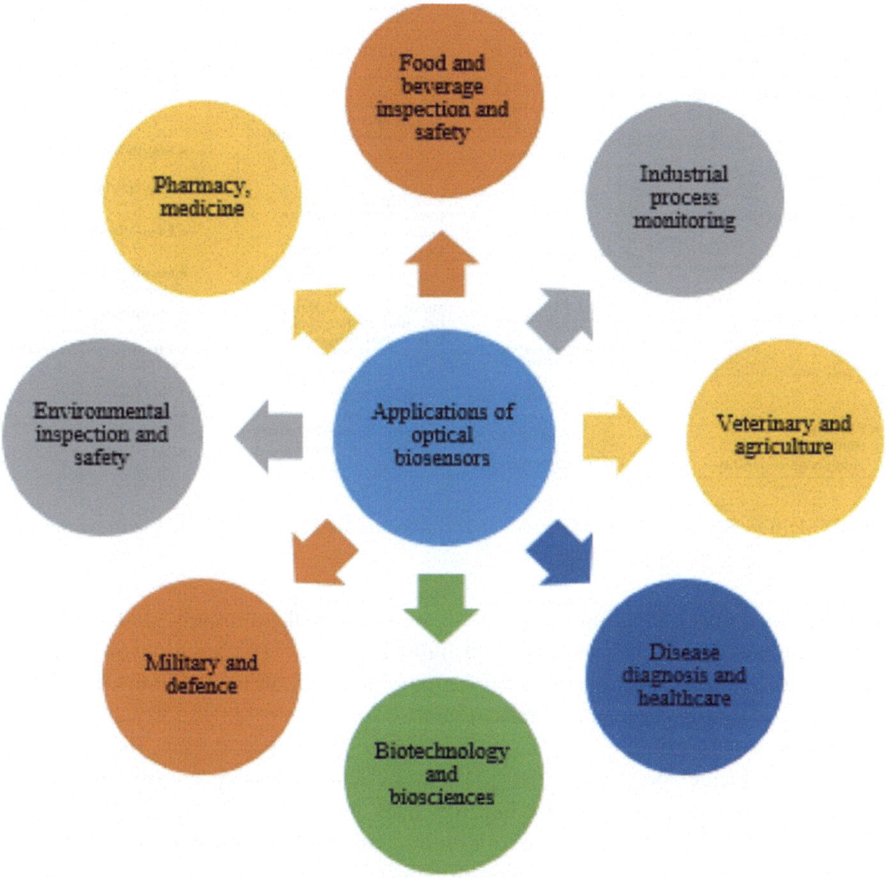

Fig. 6.2 Different applications of optical biosensor. (Adapted with permission from Ref. [42], Licence No. CC BY-NC-ND 4.0)

commonplace [49]. For instance, biosensors based on porous silicon may detect bacteria in food processing water, while low-fouling surface plasmon resonance (SPR) biosensors can detect Salmonella and Escherichia coli in food products [50–52]. The citrus disease Penicillium digitatum and the saltwater neurotoxin tetrodotoxin have both been detected using optical biosensors, which detect light reactions before the infection becomes obvious [53]. Mercury (Hg) is a prevalent water contaminant that may be detected using a cell-free optical biosensor [54–56]. This demonstrates the potential application of optical biosensors in environmental and food safety analyses.

Nanomaterials in Optical Biosensors for Contaminant Detection

Nanomaterials' (NMs) optical, electrical, physiochemical, and adsorption properties make them indispensable in the field of biosensor development [57]. Veterinary

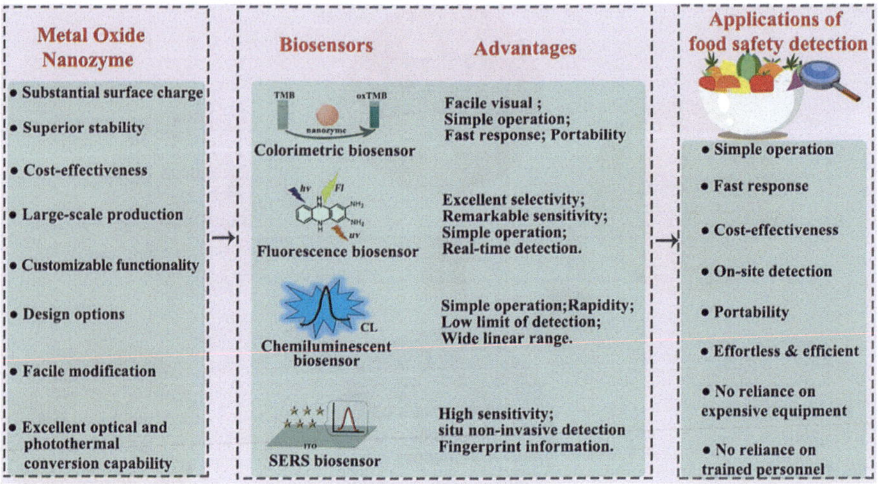

Fig. 6.3 Different type of biosensors and applications in food safety. (Adapted with permission from Ref. [44], Licence No. 6111860438491)

medication residues, pesticides, poisons, environmental pollutants, and microbiological contaminants are all readily identifiable by these characteristics [58]. Optical and electrochemical nanosensors with various transduction mechanisms have been studied for antibiotic detection. Optical nanosensors control or modify colour, surface plasmon resonance (SPR), surface-enhanced Raman scattering, fluorescence, and other electrical properties [58]. The analytical chemistry community favors fluorescence-based sensors due to their low background interference, high sensitivity, and relative ease of use. As nanoparticles bind to their antibiotic targets, these sensors detect changes in fluorescence intensity, ratiometric fluorescence output, wavelength shifts, anisotropy, and quenching [59, 60]. Ampicillin biosensors make use of luminescent nanoparticles including carbon-based nanoparticles, upconversion nanoparticles (UCNPs), quantum dots (QDs), and metal-organic frameworks (MOFs). Investigating the role of nanoparticles in the detection of fluorescence-based food antibiotic residues is covered in the next sections. Gold nanoparticles (AuNPs) have unique optical properties, are biocompatible, have excellent electrical conductivity, are inexpensive to produce, and are chemically stable, making them ideal for use in the production of fluorescent nanosensors [59, 61]. In many cases, AuNPs serve as both aptamer carriers and fluorescence quenchers. By absorbing light from organic fluorophore donors, AuNPs in FRET-based systems reduce fluorescence.

Recent research has shown that kanamycin (KMY) residue in milk may be detected using bovine serum albumin-functionalized gold nanoclusters (BSA-AuNCs) [62]. The increased fluorescence seen in hybrid materials like Au-Ag, Au-Pt, and Ag-Pt nanoparticles as a result of synergistic heteroatom interactions is a property shared by bimetallic gold nanoclusters [63]. An aptasensor for ampicillin (AMP) was developed using AuNPs linked with 3,4,9,10-perylenetetracarboxylic acid diimide (PTCDI) [64]. An aptamer-complementary strand (CS) system was used to construct the aptasensor, which was engineered to alter fluorescence intensity upon AMP binding. This successfully identifies chlortetracycline (CTC) in milk using Ag/Pt NCs@PEI, proving the versatility of AuNP-based biosensors for food safety monitoring.

For antibiotic detection, silica nanoparticles (SNPs) are an appealing nanomaterial due to their affordability, simplicity of production, hydrophilicity, and compatibility with biological systems. For the purpose of locating tetracycline (TC), Eu^{3+}-SNPs have shown to be excellent probes due to their 10 nM detection limit (LOD) [65]. A potential use for copper sulfide nanoparticles in fluorescence-based kanamycin (KMY) detection experiments is the binding of two DNA aptamer segments [66]. Toxicology, stability, and public acceptance must be considered before metallic nanoparticles may be employed in food, despite their many advantages [67–69].

As energy donors and acceptors, graphene, graphene oxide (GO), and reduced graphene oxide (rGO) are used in fluorescence-based biosensors [70]. Using these materials, energy-transfer-based detection techniques may be implemented by bringing donor and acceptor molecules close together to facilitate electron transfer and FRET [71]. In milk and eggs, β-lactamase, sulfamethazine, sulfadimethoxine, kanamycin, and AMP may be detected using aptamer-functionalized GO-based FRET biosensors [70]. Additionally, a milk aminoglycoside evanescent wave aptasensor (FQ-EWA) was developed, which employs GO as a fluorescence quencher [72]. The quenching properties of GO and enrofloxacin aptamers were used to produce a label-free fluorescence sensor and a tetracycline (TC) turn-on aptasensor. Due to GO's low background fluorescence and signal restoration upon target binding, the TC turn-on aptasensor is able to detect biological signals. Furthermore, a fluorescent nanocomposite called $BiPO_4$@GO-MMIPs was created to identify, break down, and isolate ciprofloxacin (CIP) from various materials such as milk, whole blood, and serum [72]. This method achieved a limit of detection (LOD) of 0.4 μg/L.

To improve optical probes capacity to detect target analytes in complicated mixtures, researchers have begun to use quantum dots (QDs) and molecularly imprinted polymers (MIPs) [73]. Antibiotic detection using MIP-conjugated CdTe QDs has been the focus of much investigation [74]. Sarafloxacin might be detected using a nano-aptasensor that employs CdTe QDs doped with polydopamine (PDA) and MIPs [75]. The quenching of fluorescence was proportional to the analyte concentration. Utilizing CdTe QDs, polyaniline, and graphene oxide in a MIP, the fluorescent nanocomposite sensor PANI-GOx-MIP-QDs was capable of detecting lomefloxacin [76]. A solid-state luminous sensor achieved a low limit of detection (LOD) of 0.0071 μM by using CdSe/ZnS QDs as fluorophores and SSZ-specific MIPs as recognition components. The recent progress in QD-based biosensors has opened up exciting possibilities for the development of highly sensitive and selective methods for the detection of antibiotics in many environmental and food samples.

Analytical equipment that uses paper for testing is simple, cheap, and requires very little sample size for on-site testing. A paper-based fluorescent immunoassay can detect fluorescence quantitatively by using CdTe QDs linked with anti-norfloxacin (NOR) antibodies. Antibiotic detection technology may soon include tiny and sensitive detectors built into smartphones called biosensors. A 3D-printed detection system and CdSe@SiO_2@CdTe QD hybrid fluorescent probes used in an affordable amantadine immunoassay for smartphones prove the feasibility of portable, real-time biosensing [77].

(b) **Antibiotics detection in Water**

World Health Organization (WHO) reports that environmental pathogenic bacteria are leading cause of water and food poisoning worldwide. More effective means of identification and prevention are necessary since these illnesses cause a great deal of sickness and mortality worldwide [78]. Resolving this problem is crucial for ensuring the safety of food and water throughout the globe and protecting human health. An estimated 45 million Americans fall victim to food poisoning each year, and that number is rising. As a result of the approximately 120,000 hospitalizations and 3000 deaths, the yearly economic impact amounts to $15 billion [79]. Antibiotic detection methods based on chromatography are diverse [80]. With the current setup, preparing samples is excessively time-consuming and costly. Therefore, it is more practical to develop a technique for detecting antibiotics in water that is both quick and sensitive [81]. The optical sensor takes a signal that comes from a biometric element that touches the analyte of interest and turns it into an optical signal [82]. Antibiotics are often detected using this method because to its sensitivity, ease of use, and simplicity. Optical signal transduction provides the basis for their distribution.

Fluorescent Biosensors

For environmental applications, fluorescent biosensors have gained popularity as a sensitive method to detect a variety of analytes. These biosensors are great for both quantitative and qualitative investigation of biological processes due to their high sensitivity [34, 83, 84]. Fast response, high sensitivity, and easy preparation have garnered a lot of interest for chemical sensors based on fluorescence [85]. For example, Wang et al. developed a ratiometric fluorescence point-of-care (POC) sensing platform that can detect tetracycline with a limit of detection of 10.8 nM using a smartphone [86]. The red fluorescence was produced by combining dipicolinic acid (DPA) with guanosine 5′-monophosphate disodium salt hydrate (GMP) to create an Eu-doped Ce^{+++} lanthanide fluorescent sensing material. When tetracycline is present in water samples, it blocks the energy transfer from Ce^{3+} to Eu^{3+} by coordinating with Eu^{3+}. This causes the water samples to glow blue. To avoid immobilization and/or modification processes, Tan et al. initially developed a fluorescence assay of GO hydrogels based on the target response for antibiotic detection [87]. They physically mixed GO, adenosine, and the adaptive system to prepare hydrogels, and quantitative OTC detection was achieved under mild conditions. There is some thermal and chemical stability to the hydrogel sensor as compared to the earlier technique. The range of 25 ~ 1000 μg/L is where oxytetracycline (OTC) has a linear response, and 25 μg/L is the limit of quantification. Hydrogels intended to substitute recognition elements for the detection of other compounds were also investigated by the scientists. The detection limit for fluoroquinolones was shown to be close to 50 ppb by Zhong et al., some fluoroquinolones may specifically reduce the fluorescence of MOFs in suspension [88]. The usage of a fluorescent metal-organic framework (MOF) material based on zinc (II) was described by Zhu et al. to detect sulfonamide antibiotics in the aqueous phase via the fluorescence quenching effect, thereby expanding the pH range of detection [89]. The method's versatility in handling a wide range of pH values (from 3.0 to about 9.0) and its insensitivity to heavy metal ions make it highly applicable to wastewater treatment and water quality monitoring.

Colorimetric Biosensors

Colorimetric methods have garnered interest due to their ease of preparation, speed of detection, and ability to detect significant hue shifts. Colorimetric biosensors are commonly employed to detect antibiotics in water due to their benefits [90]. Wang and coworkers developed a tetracycline colorimetric biosensor using Fe_3O_4 magnetic nanoparticles [91]. By complexing with TCs, Fe_3O_4 MNPs may increase the hydrogen peroxide oxidation of 3,3′,5,5′-tetramethylbenzidine (TMB), darkening the solution. The research findings may be observed clearly before UV-Vis spectroscopy. Under optimal circumstances, OTC had a detection limit of 26 nM, TC had 45 nM, and DOX had 48 nM. Similarly, Wang et al. designed an excellent fluorometric technique employing carbon quantum dots. Oxytetracycline (OTC) may be detected using CDs in Fe_3O_4 MNPs and H_2O_2 as a fluorescent probe [92]. Hydroxyl radicals accelerate CD fluorescence extinction. Both the CDs' excitation and OTCs' absorption bands are simultaneous. CD fluorescence is reduced by an inner filter between OTC and CDs. For OTC detection, a 9.5 nM fluorescence sensor was developed. Colorimetric biosensors function without sophisticated chemical processing, change, or experimentation. Detection and production of signals are both straightforward processes that may be accomplished with the naked eye [93].

(c) **Clinical Application for human health**

Using biosensors to identify ailments as fast as possible allows medical researchers to give health care to a large level. The use of optical transducer biosensors allows for the recording of light fluctuations that occur during the research and the interaction of biological elements [94]. This interesting attribute is explained by the biological component that is used to identify the target molecule. There is often a high degree of basicity in biological interactions, such as those between antigen-binding antibodies, enzymes and substrates, or two strands of DNA [95]. People with diabetes have the ability to control their glucose levels at home, which helps them prevent hypoglycemia. Cardiac troponin is a protein complex that indicates heart muscle damage [96]. Several commercially available devices rely on this information. An anti-troponin sensor is made use of by a biological component that is physically bound to cardiac troponin. Acute myocardial infarction is identified by medical practitioners after installing the biosensor system in a mobile unit [97, 98].

A fluorescent sensor for blood cancer detection based on GO and carboxyfluorescein-labeled Sgc8 aptamers was reported by Tan et al. GO enhances the stability of aptamers by binding to them via π-π stacking, acting as an energy receptor [99]. GO inhibited the fluorescence upon contact with a Sgc8 aptamer tagged with carboxyfluorescein when cancer cells were not present, and no signal were observed. As soon as cancer cells become accessible, the aptamer may bind to them, resulting in the production of a fluorescent signal. The fluorescence intensity is said to rise as the cell number grows. In order to detect CEA, a fluorescent sensor based on MoS_2 nanosheets and protein aptamers was created [100]. Deposition of MoS_2 nanosheets and functionalization of protein aptamers are shown schematically in Fig. 6.4. MoS_2 nanosheets are capable of initiating the transfer of energy from fluorescence resonances and have excellent quenching efficiency. A wireless biosensor that combines electrochemical sensing with fluorescence, built on polymer dot-manganese oxide complexes (PD/MnO_2), is shown to be able to identify cancer cells [101]. Interactions between polymer dots and the alkaline phosphatase found in cancer cells alter the intensity of the dots' fluorescence, that is already rather bright.

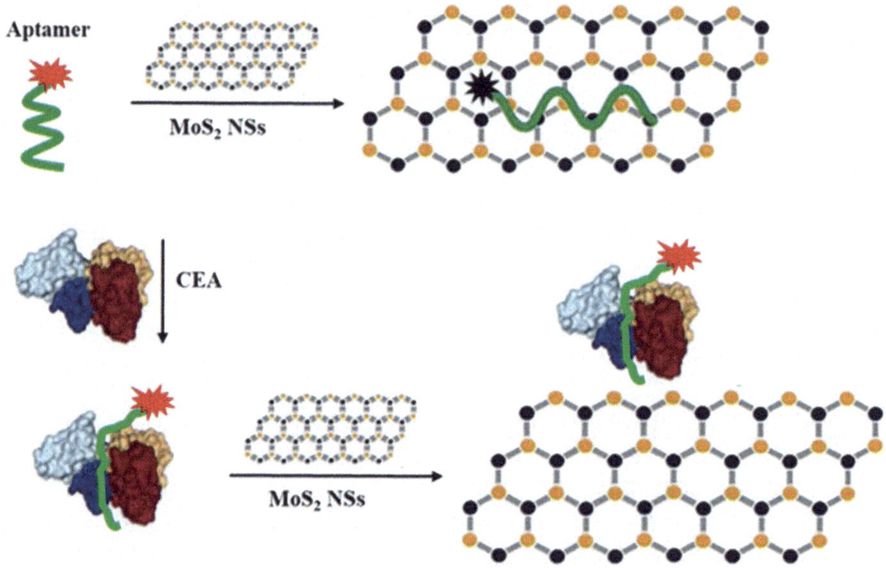

Fig. 6.4 A probe that uses aptamers and has a fluorescent dye attached to MoS_2 nanosheets. (Adapted with permission from Ref. [100], Licence No. 6111870452440)

6.4 Emerging Trends and Future Perspective:

- Antibiotic analysis and detection biosensor technology is predicted to see some fascinating developments in the future. Increased use of microfluidics and nanomaterials might render optical biosensors more sensitive to antibiotic residues in our environment. Electrochemical biosensors combined with nanomaterials like graphene may potentially provide increased sensitivity and mobility for on-site antibiotic detection. Developing multiplexed biosensor systems that can distinguish between several antibiotic classes from a single sample is one of the potentials for the future. This might be achieved by combining many aptamers or ligand binding assays on a single chip. With the advent of smartphone-based readers and wireless results transfer, antibiotic biosensors will become more widely available for rapid screening. Sample processing may be minimized using lab-on-a-chip integration and microfluidic automation.
- 2D material optical sensors based on surface plasmon resonance (SPR), fluorescence resonance energy transfer (FRET), mid-infrared, terahertz and spin-electron techniques will develop into a novel sensing platform in the future and support safety, medication administration, medical treatment, and pollution prevention and control.
- AI/ML algorithms must be involved into the design of high-performance biosensors that can handle a variety of sensing circumstances. The feature extraction procedure based on the antibiotic's detection method and the choice of suitable AI/ML techniques to reduce analysis mistakes are the two most crucial steps in the use of AI/ML algorithms. Applying interpretable AI/ML models to POCT electronic devices for multi-antibiotic detection is crucial at the same time.
- By facilitating smooth network access, the Internet of Things (IoT) has significantly advanced the development of biosensor technology, while fostering effective data transfer and remote monitoring. Rapid data collection, storage, and analysis are made possible by the integration of IoT-enabled biosensors, which increases healthcare systems' efficiency. This connection makes it easier to quickly identify abnormalities, monitor health indicators continuously, and take prompt action.
- Another promising field of future research is wearable real-time biosensors, which have many advantages, such as the ongoing evaluation of various physiological indicators that enhance our comprehension of a person's health. By enabling remote patient monitoring by medical professionals, wearable biosensors that are linked to the Internet of Things (IoT) improve the effectiveness of healthcare delivery. Those who suffer from chronic illnesses would particularly benefit from this.
- The creation of biosensors requires a team of biologists, chemists, physicists, electronics engineers, and data analytics professionals. Interdisciplinary team coordination may lead to logistical difficulties and a lack of creativity. The study focuses on integrating biosensors with digital health platforms, including mobile health apps and cloud-based data systems. Customized medicine, patient care, and diagnostics might all be revolutionized by this technology. Even though sta-

bility, repeatability, and regulatory barriers remain issues, recent advancements indicate that these technologies have a lot of promise for the future. Biosensors will become more and more significant in-patient monitoring, disease diagnosis, and healthcare delivery as their capabilities continue to develop.

6.5 Conclusion

Modern science relies on antibiotics to prevent sickness and stimulate growth. Nonetheless, they pose a threat to the ecosystem if used extensively. Constant antibiotic dosing has a negative impact on ecosystem biodiversity, which in turn has repercussions for human health. This chapter has provided an overview of the existing research on optical biosensors for detecting antibiotic residues in food, water, and healthcare facilities. The versatility to combine alternative detection algorithms, together with optical biosensors' high sensitivity and specificity, as well as their quick reaction times, have led to recent improvements in their use. Nanotechnology, advances in materials science, and improvements in data processing are driving the growing interest in optical biosensors.

Optical biosensors have been greatly improved in performance due to to the incorporation of nanomaterials like quantum dots, nanoparticles, and nanowires, which have increased their detection range and sensitivity. Based on their transduction method, optical biosensors can be categorized into many classes. These include fluorescence-based biosensors, surface plasmon resonance biosensors, fiber-optic biosensors, and nanomaterial-enhanced optical biosensors. By thoroughly examining the detection principles and construction methodologies of these sensors, we have outlined the key components and principles that characterize optical biosensors. This encompasses the Biological Recognition Element, the Optical Transduction Mechanism, and the Sensing Mechanisms. The core principles of optical biosensors focus on integrating biological recognition elements with optical transduction methods to achieve exceptional sensitivity and specificity in analyte detection. Moreover, their use in identifying antibiotic residue, medical diagnostics, and environmental monitoring underscores their crucial importance in contemporary analytical science.

The realm of optical biosensors for detecting antibiotic residues represents a dynamic area within analytical science. Nonetheless, ongoing innovation and committed research endeavors are essential to overcome existing obstacles and completely leverage the capabilities of these promising technologies. This promising path indicates a bright future, a sign of a new age of swift, effective, and easily accessible detection of antibiotic residues.

References

1. Banyal R, Sonu S, Soni V, Chawla A, Raizada P, Ahamad T et al (2024) Synergetic photocatalytic degradation of the tetracycline antibiotic over S-scheme based BiOBr/CuInS2/WO3 ternary heterojunction photocatalyst. Solid State Sci 157:107700
2. Organization WH (2011) Tackling antibiotic resistance from a food safety perspective in Europe: World Health Organization. Regional Office for Europe

3. Levy SB, Marshall B (2004) Antibacterial resistance worldwide: causes, challenges and responses. Nat Med 10(Suppl 12):S122–S1S9
4. Crooks SR, McCarney B, Traynor IM, Thompson CS, Floyd S, Elliott CT (2003) Detection of levamisole residues in bovine liver and milk by immunobiosensor. Anal Chim Acta 483(1–2):181–186
5. Hlabangana L, Memeza S (2018) Ion-pair isocratic simultaneous determination of broad spectrum antibiotics in environmental samples by HPLC with UV detection. Environ Nanotechnol Monitor Manag 10:104–111
6. Irkham I, Ibrahim AU, Pwavodi PC, Al-Turjman F, Hartati YW (2023) Smart graphene-based electrochemical nanobiosensor for clinical diagnosis. Sensors 23(4):2240
7. Thévenot DR, Toth K, Durst RA, Wilson GS (2001) Electrochemical biosensors: recommended definitions and classification. Biosens Bioelectron 16(1–2):121–131
8. Moon J, Kim G, Park SB, Lim J, Mo C (2015) Comparison of whole-cell SELEX methods for the identification of Staphylococcus aureus-specific DNA aptamers. Sensors 15(4):8884–8897
9. Majdinasab M, Hayat A, Marty JL (2018) Aptamer-based assays and aptasensors for detection of pathogenic bacteria in food samples. TrAC Trends Anal Chem 107:60–77
10. Majdinasab M, Mishra RK, Tang X, Marty JL (2020) Detection of antibiotics in food: new achievements in the development of biosensors. TrAC Trends Anal Chem 127:115883
11. Koyun A, Ahlatcolu E, Koca Y, Kara S (2012) Biosensors and their principles. A roadmap of biomedical engineers and milestones. 5:42–117
12. Chen C, Wang J (2020) Optical biosensors: an exhaustive and comprehensive review. Analyst 145(5):1605–1628
13. Kaur H, Bhosale A, Shrivastav S (2018) Biosensors: classification, fundamental characterization and new trends: a review. Int J Health Sci Res 8(6):315–333
14. Chaudhary V, Gaur P, Rustagi S (2024) Sensors, society, and sustainability. Sustain Mater Technol 40:e00952
15. Liu X, Huang D, Lai C, Zeng G, Qin L, Zhang C et al (2018) Recent advances in sensors for tetracycline antibiotics and their applications. TrAC Trends Anal Chem 109:260–274
16. Hirata E, Kiyokawa E (2016) Future perspective of single-molecule FRET biosensors and intravital FRET microscopy. Biophys J 111(6):1103–1111
17. Geng Y, Guo M, Tan J, Huang S, Tang Y, Tan L et al (2018) A fluorescent molecularly imprinted polymer using aptamer as a functional monomer for sensing of kanamycin. Sensors Actuators B Chem 268:47–54
18. Fernández F, Sánchez-Baeza F, Marco M-P (2012) Nanogold probe enhanced surface plasmon resonance immunosensor for improved detection of antibiotic residues. Biosens Bioelectron 34(1):151–158
19. Situ C, Mooney MH, Elliott CT, Buijs J (2010) Advances in surface plasmon resonance biosensor technology towards high-throughput, food-safety analysis. TrAC Trends Anal Chem 29(11):1305–1315
20. Chand S, Gupta B (2007) Surface plasmon resonance based fiber-optic sensor for the detection of pesticide. Sensors Actuators B Chem 123(2):661–666
21. Homola J (2003) Present and future of surface plasmon resonance biosensors. Anal Bioanal Chem 377:528–539
22. Leung A, Shankar PM, Mutharasan R (2007) A review of fiber-optic biosensors. Sensors Actuators B Chem 125(2):688–703
23. Mehrvar M, Bis C, Scharer JM, Moo-Young M, Luong JH (2000) Fiber-optic biosensors-trends and advances. Anal Sci 16(7):677–692
24. Gong Z, Chan HT, Chen Q, Chen H (2021) Application of nanotechnology in analysis and removal of heavy metals in food and water resources. Nano 11(7):1792
25. Fondjo FF (2018) Development of nanomaterial based sensors for biomedical applications. Washington State University
26. Azab MY, Hameed MFO, Obayya SS (2023) Overview of optical biosensors for early cancer detection: fundamentals, applications and future perspectives. Biology 12(2):232

27. Kaur B, Kumar S, Nedoma J, Martinek R, Marques C (2024) Advancements in optical biosensing techniques: from fundamentals to future prospects. APL Photonics 9(9)
28. Rizwan M, Mohd-Naim NF, Ahmed MU (2018) Trends and advances in electrochemiluminescence nanobiosensors. Sensors 18(1):166
29. Khansili N, Rattu G, Krishna PM (2018) Label-free optical biosensors for food and biological sensor applications. Sensors Actuators B Chem 265:35–49
30. Kaur J, Singh PK (2020) Enzyme-based optical biosensors for organophosphate class of pesticide detection. Phys Chem Chem Phys 22(27):15105–15119
31. Yildirim N, Long F, Gao C, He M, Shi H-C, Gu AZ (2012) Aptamer-based optical biosensor for rapid and sensitive detection of 17β-estradiol in water samples. Environ Sci Technol 46(6):3288–3294
32. Monk DJ, Walt DR (2004) Optical fiber-based biosensors. Anal Bioanal Chem 379:931–945
33. Yang F, Ma Y, Stanciu SG, Wu A (2020) Transduction process-based classification of biosensors. In: Nanobiosensors: From Design to Applications, pp 23–44
34. Strianese M, Staiano M, Ruggiero G, Labella T, Pellecchia C, D'Auria S (2012) Fluorescence-based biosensors. In: Spectroscopic methods of analysis: methods and protocols, pp 193–216
35. Zhao Y, Tong R-j, Xia F, Peng Y (2019) Current status of optical fiber biosensor based on surface plasmon resonance. Biosens Bioelectron 142:111505
36. Campbell DP, McCloskey CJ (2002) Interferometric biosensors. In: Optical Biosensors. Elsevier, pp 277–304
37. Notingher I (2007) Raman spectroscopy cell-based biosensors. Sensors 7(8):1343–1358
38. Shi Y, Zhou Q, Dong S, Zhao Q, Wu X, Yang P et al (2024) Rapid, visual, label-based biosensor platform for identification of hepatitis C virus in clinical applications. BMC Microbiol 24(1):68
39. Cao J, Tu MH, Sun T, Grattan KT (2013) Wavelength-based localized surface plasmon resonance optical fiber biosensor. Sensors Actuators B Chem 181:611–619
40. Rasmi Y, Li X, Khan J, Ozer T, Choi JR (2021) Emerging point-of-care biosensors for rapid diagnosis of COVID-19: current progress, challenges, and future prospects. Anal Bioanal Chem 413(16):4137–4159
41. Neethirajan S, Ragavan K, Weng X (2018) Agro-defense: biosensors for food from healthy crops and animals. Trends Food Sci Technol 73:25–44
42. Singh AK, Mittal S, Das M, Saharia A, Tiwari M (2023) Optical biosensors: a decade in review. Alex Eng J 67:673–691
43. Markandan K, Tiong YW, Sankaran R, Subramanian S, Markandan UD, Chaudhary V et al (2024) Emergence of infectious diseases and role of advanced nanomaterials in point-of-care diagnostics: a review. Biotechnol Genet Eng Rev 40(4):3438–3526
44. Qin J, Guo N, Yang J, Wei J (2024) Recent advances in metal oxide nanozyme-based optical biosensors for food safety assays. Food Chem 447:139019
45. Wang Y, Jia K, Lin J (2024) Optical biosensors for the detection of foodborne pathogens: recent development and future prospects. TrAC Trends Anal Chem 177:117785
46. Damathia B, Pathania D, Jha A, Sable H, Singh P, Singh V et al (2025) Emergence of potassium solubilizing microbes-assisted crop processing for sustainable food production and microbial complexities. Food Bioprod Process
47. Abedi-Firoozjah R, Ebdali H, Soltani M, Abdolahi-Fard P, Heydari M, Assadpour E et al (2024) Nanomaterial-based sensors for the detection of pathogens and microbial toxins in the food industry; a review on recent progress. Coord Chem Rev 500:215545
48. Luo Y, Sun Y, Wei X, He Y, Wang H, Cui Z et al (2024) Detection methods for antibiotics in wastewater: a review. Bioprocess Biosyst Eng 47(9):1433–1451
49. Ibrahim F, Babaniyi GG, Ajao BH, Akor UJ, Daramola OE Current trends and future research in emerging food contaminants. In: Emerging contaminants in food and food products. CRC Press, pp 251–268
50. Singh L, Sharanagat VS (2024) Application of biosensors against food-borne pathogens. Nutr Food Sci 54(1):207–237

51. Forinová M, Pilipenco A, Lynn NS, Obořilová R, Šimečková H, Vrabcová M et al (2024) A reusable QCM biosensor with stable antifouling nano-coating for on-site reagent-free rapid detection of E. coli O157: H7 in food products. Food Control 165:110695
52. Sable H, Kumar V, Singh V, Rustagi S, Chahal S, Chaudhary V (2024) Strategically engineering advanced nanomaterials for heavy-metal remediation from wastewater. Coord Chem Rev 518:216079
53. Ahuja V, Singh A, Paul D, Dasgupta D, Urajová P, Ghosh S et al (2023) Recent advances in the detection of food toxins using mass spectrometry. Chem Res Toxicol 36(12):1834–1863
54. Kannappan S, Ramisetty BCM (2022) Engineered whole-cell-based biosensors: sensing environmental heavy metal pollutants in water—a review. Appl Biochem Biotechnol 194:1–27
55. Gupta S, Sarkar S, Katranidis A, Bhattacharya J (2019) Development of a cell-free optical biosensor for detection of a broad range of mercury contaminants in water: a plasmid DNA-based approach. ACS Omega 4(5):9480–9487
56. Chaudhary V, Sonu S, Taha BA, Raizada P, Rustagi S, Chahal S et al (2025) Borophene-based nanomaterials: promising candidates for next-generation gas/vapor chemiresistors. J Mater Sci Technol 218:236–262
57. Alsaiari NS, Katubi KMM, Alzahrani FM, Siddeeg SM, Tahoon MA (2021) The application of nanomaterials for the electrochemical detection of antibiotics: a review. Micromachines 12(3):308
58. Dongare PR, Gore AH (2021) Recent advances in colorimetric and fluorescent chemosensors for ionic species: design, principle and optical signalling mechanism. Chem Select 6(23):5657–5669
59. Singh H, Thakur B, Bhardwaj SK, Khatri M, Kim K-H, Bhardwaj N (2023) Nanomaterial-based fluorescent biosensors for the detection of antibiotics in foodstuffs: a review. Food Chem 426:136657
60. Chauhan N, Sankhla MS, Sharma A, Sable H, Sharma T (2025) Nanotechnology-enhanced detection of illicit drugs: development of nano sensors for rapid identification in liquid media. J Electrochem Society 172:077505
61. Sable H, Kumar V, Singh V, Rustagi S, Chaudhary V, Pandit S (2024) Nanosystems-enhanced electrochemical biosensors for precision in one health management. J Electrochem Soc 171(3):037527
62. Geng Y, Zhang S, Wang Y, Ye N, Xiang Y (2021) Aptamer act as fluorescence switching of bovine serum albumin stabilized gold nanoclusters for ultrasensitive detection of kanamycin in milk. Microchem J 165:106145
63. Xu N, Meng L, Li H-W, Lu D-Y, Wu Y (2018) Polyethyleneimine capped bimetallic Au/Pt nanoclusters are a viable fluorescent probe for specific recognition of chlortetracycline among other tetracycline antibiotics. Microchim Acta 185:1–8
64. Esmaelpourfarkhani M, Abnous K, Taghdisi SM, Chamsaz M (2020) A novel turn-off fluorescent aptasensor for ampicillin detection based on perylenetetracarboxylic acid diimide and gold nanoparticles. Biosens Bioelectron 164:112329
65. Zhang Z, Qaitoon A, Yong J, Xu Z, Zhang R. Development of a europium (III) ion functionalized silica Na-noprobe for highly sensitive detection of tetracycline. 2021
66. Belal AS, Ismail A, Elnaggar MM, Belal TS (2018) Click chemistry inspired copper sulphide nanoparticle-based fluorescence assay of kanamycin using DNA aptamer. Spectrochim Acta A Mol Biomol Spectrosc 205:48–54
67. Kaur J, Singh H, Khatri M (2020) Regulatory considerations for safety of nanomaterials. In: Nanomedicine for bioactives: Healthcare applications, pp 431–450
68. Singh V, Kasana E, Batra J, Sable H, Saxena R (2022) Antimicrobial resistance: mechanisms, screening techniques and biosensors. J Pharm Negat Results 13:1724–1735
69. Sable H, Singh V, Kumar V, Roy A, Pandit S, Kaur K et al (2024) Toxicological and bioremediation profiling of nonessential heavy metals (mercury, chromium, cadmium, aluminium) and their impact on human health: a review. Toxicologie Analytique et Clinique 36(3):205–234

70. Kou Q, Wu P, Sun Q, Li C, Zhang L, Shi H et al (2021) Selection and truncation of aptamers for ultrasensitive detection of sulfamethazine using a fluorescent biosensor based on graphene oxide. Anal Bioanal Chem 413:901–909
71. Zhou Y, Mahapatra C, Chen H, Peng X, Ramakrishna S, Nanda HS (2020) Recent developments in fluorescent aptasensors for detection of antibiotics. Curr Opin Biomed Eng 13:16–24
72. Tang Y, Gu C, Wang C, Song B, Zhou X, Lou X et al (2018) Evanescent wave aptasensor for continuous and online aminoglycoside antibiotics detection based on target binding facilitated fluorescence quenching. Biosens Bioelectron 102:646–651
73. Yang J, Lin Z-Z, Nur A-Z, Lu Y, Wu M-H, Zeng J et al (2018) Detection of trace tetracycline in fish via synchronous fluorescence quenching with carbon quantum dots coated with molecularly imprinted silica. Spectrochim Acta A Mol Biomol Spectrosc 190:450–456
74. Wang X, Zhang L, Hao A, Shi Z, Dai C, Yang Y et al (2020) Silica-coated silver nanoparticles decorated with fluorescent CdTe quantum dots and DNA aptamers for detection of tetracycline. ACS Appl Nano Mater 3(10):9796–9803
75. Chaowana R, Bunkoed O (2019) A nanocomposite probe of polydopamine/molecularly imprinted polymer/quantum dots for trace sarafloxacin detection in chicken meat. Anal Bioanal Chem 411:6081–6090
76. Orachorn N, Bunkoed O (2019) A nanocomposite fluorescent probe of polyaniline, graphene oxide and quantum dots incorporated into highly selective polymer for lomefloxacin detection. Talanta 203:261–268
77. Yu W, Jiang C, Xie B, Wang S, Yu X, Wen K et al (2020) Ratiometric fluorescent sensing system for drug residue analysis: highly sensitive immunosensor using dual-emission quantum dots hybrid and compact smartphone based-device. Anal Chim Acta 1102:91–98
78. Mohammad A-M, Chowdhury T, Biswas B, Absar N (2018) Food poisoning and intoxication: a global leading concern for human health. In: Food safety and preservation. Elsevier, pp 307–352
79. Almaary KS (2023) Food-borne diseases and their impact on health. Biosci Biotechnol Res Asia 20(3):745–755
80. Zeng Y, Chang F, Liu Q, Duan L, Li D, Zhang H (2022) Recent advances and perspectives on the sources and detection of antibiotics in aquatic environments. Journal of Analytical Methods in Chemistry 2022(1):5091181
81. Nehra M, Dilbaghi N, Kumar R, Kumar S (2022) Trends in point-of-care optical biosensors for antibiotics detection in aqueous media. Mater Lett 308:131235
82. Han F, Wang T, Liu G, Liu H, Xie X, Wei Z et al (2022) Materials with tunable optical properties for wearable epidermal sensing in health monitoring. Adv Mater 34(26):2109055
83. Girigoswami K, Akhtar N (2019) Nanobiosensors and fluorescence based biosensors: an overview. Int J Nano Dimension 10(1):1–17
84. Sable H, Singh V, Khosla A, Chaudhary V (2025) Detection and analysis of cadmium prevalence in soil-water matrices of industrial settings of Delhi: bioavailability and geochemical study. J Electrochem Soc 172(2):027514
85. Guo L, Yang L, Li M, Kuang L, Song Y, Wang L (2021) Covalent organic frameworks for fluorescent sensing: recent developments and future challenges. Coord Chem Rev 440:213957
86. Wang T, Mei Q, Tao Z, Wu H, Zhao M, Wang S et al (2020) A smartphone-integrated ratiometric fluorescence sensing platform for visual and quantitative point-of-care testing of tetracycline. Biosens Bioelectron 148:111791
87. Tan B, Zhao H, Du L, Gan X, Quan X (2016) A versatile fluorescent biosensor based on target-responsive graphene oxide hydrogel for antibiotic detection. Biosens Bioelectron 83:267–273
88. Zhong W-B, Li R-X, Lv J, He T, Xu M-M, Wang B et al (2020) Two isomeric In (III)-MOFs: unexpected stability difference and selective fluorescence detection of fluoroquinolone antibiotics in water. Inorganic Chem Front 7(5):1161–1171
89. Zhu X-D, Zhang K, Wang Y, Long W-W, Sa R-J, Liu T-F et al (2018) Fluorescent metal–organic framework (MOF) as a highly sensitive and quickly responsive chemical sensor for the detection of antibiotics in simulated wastewater. Inorg Chem 57(3):1060–1065

90. Zhou Y, Huang X, Hu X, Tong W, Leng Y, Xiong Y (2021) Recent advances in colorimetry/fluorimetry-based dual-modal sensing technologies. Biosens Bioelectron 190:113386
91. Wang Y, Sun Y, Dai H, Ni P, Jiang S, Lu W et al (2016) A colorimetric biosensor using Fe3O4 nanoparticles for highly sensitive and selective detection of tetracyclines. Sensors Actuators B Chem 236:621–626
92. Wang L, Zhou H, Wu X, Song Y, Huang Y, Yang X et al (2022) A novel colorimetric aptasensor for sensitive tetracycline detection based on the peroxidase-like activity of Fe3O4@Cu nanoparticles and "sandwich" oligonucleotide hybridization. Microchim Acta 189(3):86
93. Sumitha M, Xavier T (2023) Recent advances in electrochemical biosensors–a brief review. Hybrid Advances 2:100023
94. Kaur B, Kumar S, Kaushik BK (2022) Recent advancements in optical biosensors for cancer detection. Biosens Bioelectron 197:113805
95. Uniyal A, Srivastava G, Pal A, Taya S, Muduli A (2023) Recent advances in optical biosensors for sensing applications: a review. Plasmonics 18(2):735–750
96. Pourali A, Rashidi MR, Barar J, Pavon-Djavid G, Omidi Y (2021) Voltammetric biosensors for analytical detection of cardiac troponin biomarkers in acute myocardial infarction. TrAC Trends Anal Chem 134:116123
97. Kim SY, Lee J-P, Shin W-R, Oh I-H, Ahn J-Y, Kim Y-H (2022) Cardiac biomarkers and detection methods for myocardial infarction. Mol Cell Toxicol 18(4):443–455
98. Chaudhary V, Lucky L, Sable H, Bhalla N (2025) Interdisciplinary approach to Monkeypox prevention: integrating nanobiosensors, nanovaccines, artificial intelligence, visual arts, and social sciences. Small Struct 6:2400647
99. Tan J, Lai Z, Zhong L, Zhang Z, Zheng R, Su J et al (2018) A graphene oxide-based fluorescent aptasensor for the turn-on detection of CCRF-CEM. Nanoscale Res Lett 13:1–8
100. Zhao L, Cheng M, Liu G, Lu H, Gao Y, Yan X et al (2018) A fluorescent biosensor based on molybdenum disulfide nanosheets and protein aptamer for sensitive detection of carcinoembryonic antigen. Sensors Actuators B Chem 273:185–190
101. Won HJ, Robby AI, Jhon HS, In I, Ryu JH, Park SY (2020) Wireless label-free electrochemical detection of cancer cells by MnO2-decorated polymer dots. Sensors Actuators B Chem 320:128391

Advanced Point-of-Care Biosensors Integrated with AI and Bioinformatics

7

Bakr Ahmed Taha, Ali J. Addie, Adawiya J. Haider, and Norhana Arsad

7.1 Introduction

Point-of-care (POC) biosensors constitute a transformative improvement in contemporary healthcare, allowing speedy and accurate analysis without delay at the point of care. These instruments are mainly vital in chronic sicknesses and powerful control of infectious conditions, as they facilitate timely scientific intervention that could enhance affected person results and fine of existence. Integrating biosensors into POC testing, in particular the need for fast diagnostic abilities, has been highlighted all through the COVID-19 pandemic, which has been proving vital to preventing infection at the threshold [1–6]. Transduction methods of biosensors include electrochemical, optical, and piezoelectric [7–9]. Electrochemical biosensors are especially attractive due to their portability and cost-effectiveness, enabling them to

B. A. Taha (✉)
Photonics Technology Lab, Department of Electrical, Electronic and Systems Engineering, Faculty of Engineering and Built Environment, Universiti Kebangsaan Malaysia, UKM, Bangi, Malaysia

Al-imam University College, Balad, Iraq
e-mail: dra@ukm.edu.my

A. J. Addie
Center of Industrial Applications and Materials Technology, Scientific Research Commission, Baghdad, Iraq

A. J. Haider
Applied Sciences Department/Laser Science and Technology Branch, University of Technology, Baghdad, Iraq

N. Arsad
Photonics Technology Lab, Department of Electrical, Electronic and Systems Engineering, Faculty of Engineering and Built Environment, Universiti Kebangsaan Malaysia, UKM, Bangi, Malaysia
e-mail: noa@ukm.edu.my

V. Chaudhary, N. Bhalla (eds.), *Biosensors for Tackling Antimicrobial Resistance (AMR)*, https://doi.org/10.1007/978-981-95-9151-0_7

be integrated with mobile devices such as smartphones. Smartphone-based diagnostic systems that use advanced imaging techniques to determine the results of lateral flow assays (LFAS) represent this trend. The development of such innovations increases the purpose of POC units, which can be used in different fields, including environmental monitoring and food security [10–14].

Thus, POC biosensors can only be used for tracking non-stop persistent conditions, including diabetes and heart disease [15]. Healthcare professionals can use these units to create knowledgeable alternatives based on real-time registers, improve treatment efficiency, and monitor patients. Nanostructures and polymers have also made it possible to develop special touch and selective biosensors for detecting low biomarker concentrations. This functionality is important for detecting early illness, where a well-door of time-bound disease can significantly adjust disease growth and handling techniques [16–18].

Integrating artificial intelligence (AI) and bioinformatics in biosensor generations is desirable because of the possibilities and packages of these things in different fields, especially in health and environmental tracking. This synthesis suggests how these technologies have coordinated to increase the biosphere's performance, sensitivity and uniqueness. AI, especially System Study (ML), is important for promoting biosensor technology. Recent research states that ML technology can adapt to biosensor wording and analysis methods to explain complex characters more effectively. A department for AI applies quickly to data analysis in chemometrics biosensors and increases its clinical capabilities [19–22]. Furthermore, ML has been instrumental in developing high-normal overall performance electrochemical sensors, demonstrating its versatility at some point in high-quality biosensing programs [23]. The functionality of ML to device large datasets allows for the identification of styles and anomalies that conventional methods might also neglect, for this reason, improving the reliability of biosensors in clinical and environmental setting [24]. Bioinformatics supports AI by providing computational gear to lay out and optimize biosensors. Structural bioinformatics can discover allosteric sites in a protein, facilitating the insertion of sensor domain names that beautify biosensor applications. Furthermore, bioinformatics tools assist in directing the evolution of proteins, enabling researchers to explore mutational situations that can lead to enhanced sensor properties [25–27]. Furthermore, combining AI and bioinformatics ends in personalized remedies via wearable biosensors. These devices can screen physiological alerts in real-time, using AI algorithms to provide insights into character health fame. The capacity of AI-powered biosensors to facilitate factor-of-care diagnosis is especially promising, as it can provide timely and accurate fitness exams, thereby enhancing patient outcomes. Wearable biosensors have been designed to mechanically detect opioid intake, demonstrating the realistic position of AI in monitoring drug use and promoting public health [28, 29].

7.2 Fundamentals of Point-of-Care Biosensors

Biosensors are analytical devices that convert biological responses into electrical signals, enabling the detection of various chemical compounds in nature. The definition of biosensors encompasses a wide range of systems in which biological agents, such as enzymes, antibodies, or whole cells, are used to detect the conversion of specific analytes into measurable signals, and multidisciplinary biosensor combines biological chemical and engineering principles [30]. There are three types of biosensors: biosensors, conversion methods, and application sites. Among the most used biosensors are enzymatic biosensors, which catalyze specific reactions with target analytes using enzymes. A cell-based biosensor detects environmental changes or specific parameters using living cells, and immunosensors detect proteins and pathogens using antibody-antigen interactions [31–33].

Concerning conversion methods, biosensors are classified electrically, detecting changes in electrical conductivity arising from biochemical reactions; optical, which relates to photointeractions such as fluorescence for analyte detection; and mass sensitive, measuring the change in mass upon analyte binding. In applications, biosensors are used for medical research to detect diseases and monitor health, environmental monitoring to detect pollution and toxicity, and food safety to detect contaminants or indications things are ruined. This combination of AI and biosensors is especially useful at the point of care. This combination of AI and biosensors will lead to smarter, more efficient diagnostic tools that provide real-time health monitoring and decision support [34–37]. An enzyme or antibody interacting with a target analyte is referred to as a biosensor, and the transducer converts this interaction into a measurable signal; the signal processing unit amplifies and processes the signal, and the output display shows the results, as shown in Fig. 7.1. Moreover, radiometric methods are effective for the detection and measurement of analytes. This method requires

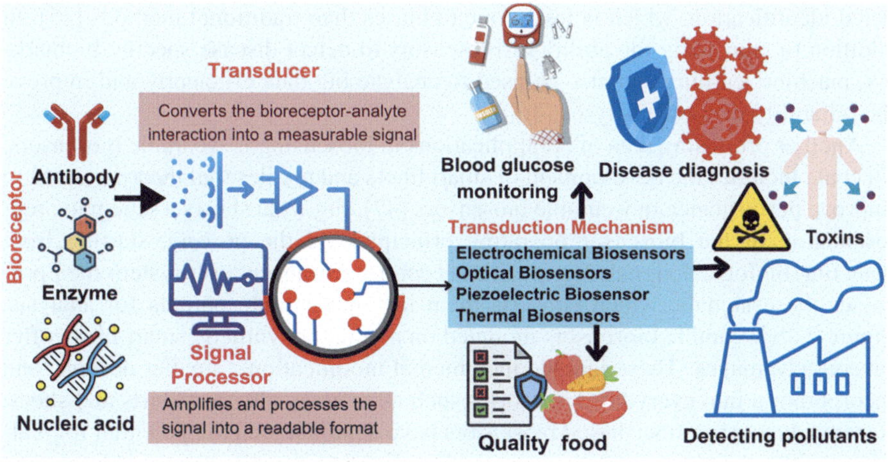

Fig. 7.1 Represents the functionality of a biosensor

monitoring changes in the ratio of two or more signals to maximize accuracy and sensitivity. Ratio measurement methods have been widely used in medical research, environmental monitoring, and food safety. They are particularly useful when single signal detection methods are not practical, and these methods are well suited for analyte detection under complex conditions by providing improved accuracy and reliability, especially when materials the presence of distractions that can impair accuracy. The article [38], focuses on ratiometric fluorescent nanoprobes for visual analyte detection. Development of two-photon fluorescence probes for biomedical imaging, synthesis of ratiometric surface-enhanced Raman scattering nanoprobes for intracellular analyzer imaging, molecularly imprinted electrochemical sensors for detection of electroactive species, and matrices—Auxiliary laser desorption/ionization for ratiometric probes. Each method is described in detail, and its principles, advantages, applications, and limitations are discussed.

7.3 Integration of Artificial Intelligence in Biosensing

Diagnostics and health monitoring require the application of artificial intelligence (AI) in biosensing technologies, which improves biosensor performance by increasing sensitivity, specificity, and data processing, leading to more accurate and timely health assessments. A notable application is the development of advanced biosensors for rapid disease detection [39–42]. Tokpah and others highlight the need for decentralized, point-of-care diagnostic tools that integrate biosensors and AI and provide faster and higher yields, especially for infectious diseases such as COVID-19 [43]. Similarly, Zhang describes how AI-driven algorithms can analyze complex data from multi-parameter biosensors for more accurate food contamination detection [44]. This integration supports real-time monitoring and decision-making, which is important in a clinical environment. Machine learning (ML) techniques are also changing the interpretation of biosensor data. Jin notes that ML facilitates unlabeled identification, which is less prone to biases than traditional methods [45]. In addition to enhancing the ability of biosensors to detect disease-specific biomarkers, machine learning can also be used to analyze big data efficiently and improve the reliability of those analyses [46].

Another promising area of AI applications in biosensing is wearable biosensors. Fu et al., includes the development of smart fibers and textiles that incorporate AI to improve performance in wearable biosensors [47], Fig. 7.2a shows a schematic representation of the biosensor operating principle and the process, starting from detecting biological signals by specific receptors. A transduction system then processes these signals, which converts them into measurable outputs for analysis. Figure 7.2b Wearable biosensors mounted on natural or synthetic smart fibers offer several advantages. These include incremental modifications, smaller designs, and incorporation into everyday accessories such as scarves, gloves, t-shirts and shoes. Recent advances in fiber-based biosensors have demonstrated the potential for real-time health monitoring and environmental sensing to be easily integrated into wearable industrial systems, making them feasible to use in various ways. These

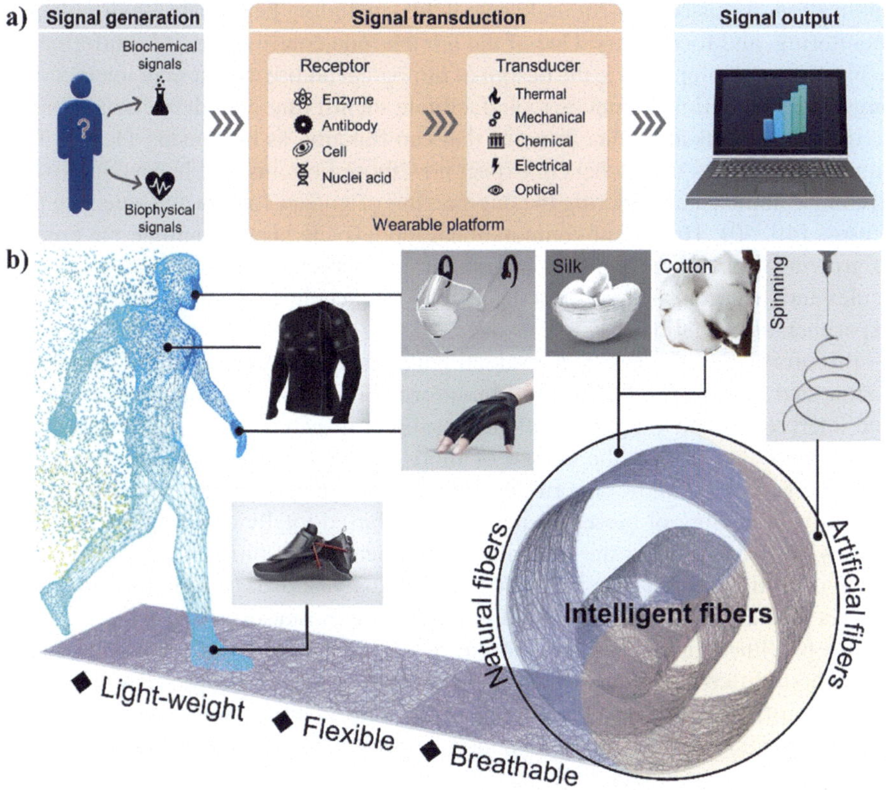

Fig. 7.2 (**a**) Schematic illustration of biosensor concepts: Receivers detect biosignals, which are then transformed into measurables. (**b**) Fiber-based wearable biosensors highlight the advantages of natural and synthetic fibers in applications such as masks, gloves, and clothing monitors. (Reprinted and permission from [47], Copyright 2024, Responsive Materials)

innovations improve sensing performance and enable seamless integration of wireless communication technologies, enabling continuous health monitoring. AI algorithms have provided real-time information and personalized healthcare solutions to chronic diseases, including diabetes [48]. Furthermore, the use of AI in biosensing extends to the food industry, where it helps detect antibiotic residues and contaminants. Lu notes that AI-powered biosensors can process large amounts of sensing data, improving the detection of many food antibiotics. This capability is important for food safety and health regulation if they are obeyed.

7.4 Role of Bioinformatics in Biosensor Development

Bioinformatics plays a critical role in improving biosensors, which are analytical devices that convert organic responses into measurable signals. Integrating bioinformatics into biosensor improvement complements the layout, optimization, and application of this equipment in diverse fields, including healthcare, environmental monitoring, and food safety. One of the number one contribution of bioinformatics to biosensor development is the design of biological additives that may interact with target analytes. Bioinformatics tools facilitate identifying and characterizing transcription elements and other proteins that can function as biosensing factors. This equipment permits researchers to expect how those proteins will behave in distinctive environments, considering the engineering of greater touchy and selective biosensors [49, 50]. The use of computational models can also streamline the process of growing biosensors by means of simulating interactions among biological molecules and their goals, which can considerably reduce the time and assets wished for experimental validation [51, 52].

Bioinformatics also assists in evaluating big datasets generated during biosensor testing and optimization. Advanced bioinformatics software programs can system and interpret complex organic statistics, enabling researchers to identify styles and correlations that inform the design of more effective biosensors. The mixing of machine-getting-to-know algorithms into bioinformatics workflows permits the predictive modeling of biosensor performance-based totally on historical information, which can beautify the reliability and efficiency of biosensor programs [53, 54]. In addition to assisting in the design and analysis phases, bioinformatics also plays a pivotal role in validating and standardizing biosensors. Improving bioinformatics pipelines guarantees that biosensor facts are reproducible and comparable throughout different studies, which is essential for regulatory approval and medical utility. Furthermore, bioinformatics tools can help identify biomarkers, which are essential for improving biosensors aimed at specific diseases, along with most cancers or infectious sicknesses [55–57].

The application of bioinformatics in biosensor development is exemplified by a variety of studies that have successfully integrated these approaches. Using bioinformatics to design DNA-based biosensors has led to developing highly sensitive tools for detecting specific nucleic acid sequences, which can be used to diagnose infectious diseases [58, 59]. Similarly, bioinformatics contributes to developing electrochemical biosensors using nanomaterials, increasing their sensitivity and specificity for detecting low-abundance biomarkers [60–63].

In conclusion, bioinformatics is an important part of biosensor development, providing the tools and techniques needed to optimize, optimize, and validate these analytical devices. As biosensor technology evolves, bioinformatics integration will lead to even more sophisticated and effective biosensing solutions. Researchers have discussed that protein-protein ligand interaction is broadly employed in nanobiosensors because of the unique docking among unique 3D systems, making it an effective tool in bioanalysis and nanodiagnostics. These sensors permit speedy, cost-effective, touchy, and precise detection of molecular biomarkers in actual samples. Their effectiveness stems from the specific conformations of proteins; however, demanding situations such as low docking performance and difficulties in fixation on foundational layers persist. To deal with these troubles, developers optimize protein shape and features using nanoscale calculations facilitated using bioinformatics tools. This article affords a top-level view of how these gears guide

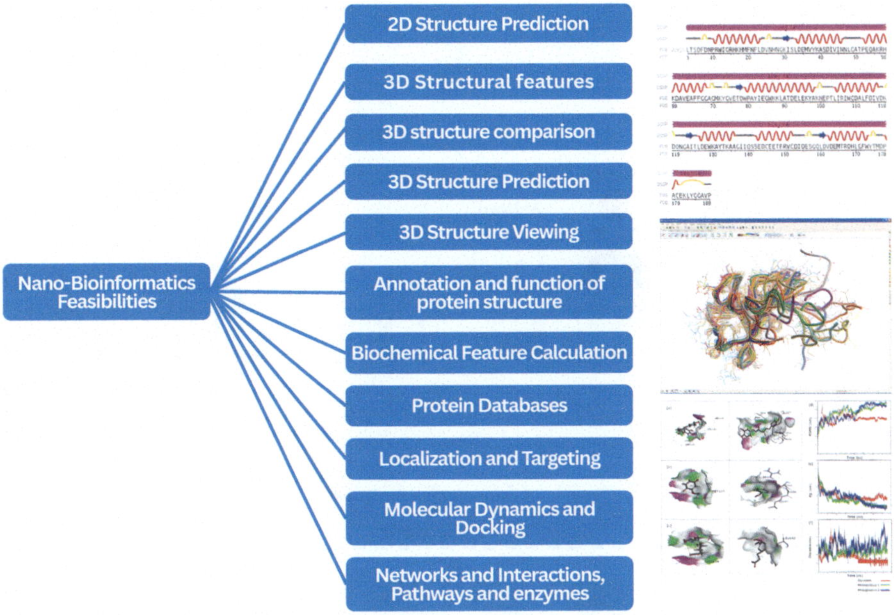

Fig. 7.3 demonstrates molecular diagnostics based on protein docking analysis combined with bioinformatics tools, providing a highly sensitive and quantitative method for diagnosing infectious diseases such as SARS-CoV-2. This combination contributes to the development of highly sensitive nano-biosensor technologies. (Reprinted and permission from [64], Copyright 2021, Biochemistry and Biophysics Reports)

modeling and optimizing the physiochemical properties of proteins on the nanoscale [64] as shown in Fig. 7.3.

7.5 Hybrid Nanomaterials in Biosensor Design

Hybrid nanomaterials have emerged as a pivotal element in designing and growing superior biosensors, leveraging their residences to enhance sensitivity, selectivity, and capability. These materials, which combine natural and inorganic factors on the nanoscale, provide a synergistic impact that may appreciably improve the overall performance of biosensing structures. Integrating hybrid nanomaterials into biosensor layout allows for exploiting their numerous houses. For example, steel-natural frameworks (MOFs) blended with carbon nanofibers have established more desirable gasoline sensitivity, showcasing the capacity of hybrid systems in gas sensing programs [65]. Similarly, the combination of steel oxides with graphene and carbon nanotubes has led to biosensors with superior optical, magnetic, and electrical properties, allowing the detection of biomolecules with high precision [66], see Fig. 7.4a. These advancements highlight the versatility of hybrid nanomaterials in tailoring sensor responses to specific analytes.

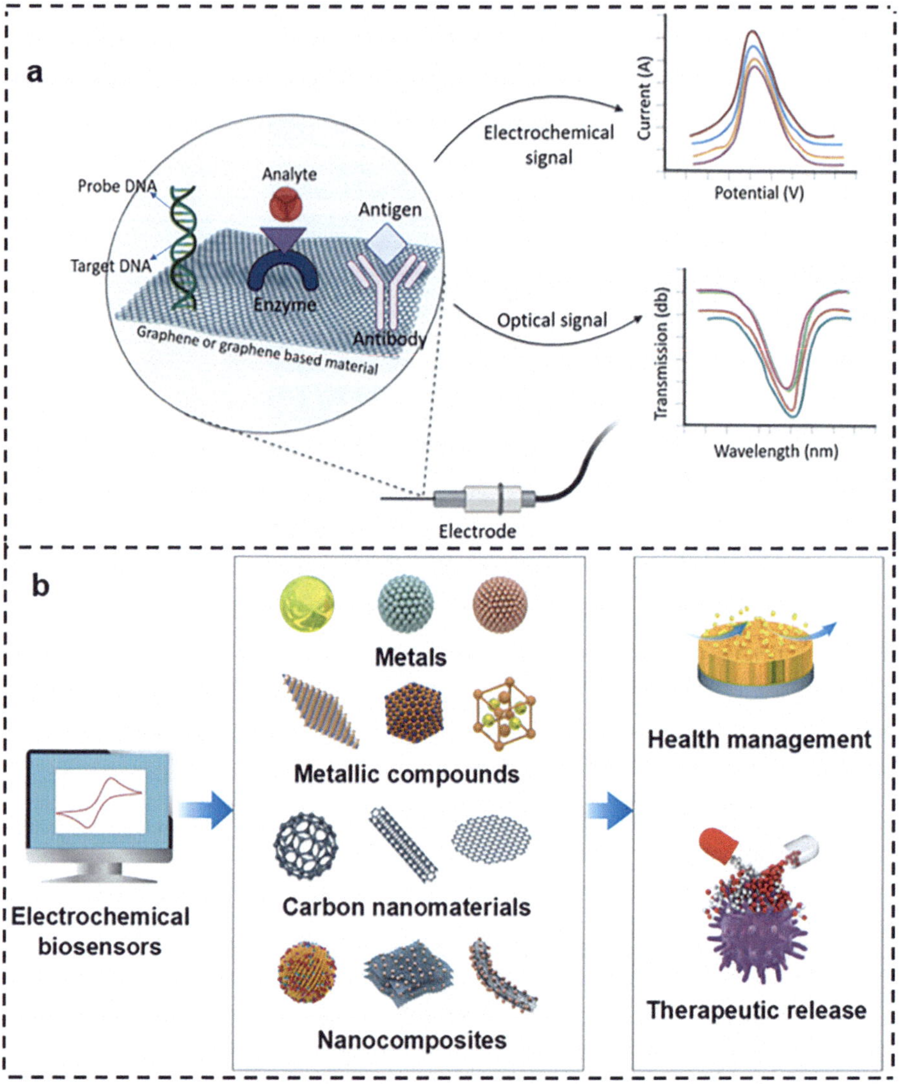

Fig. 7.4 (**a**) Graphene-based biosensors and their mechanism. (Reprinted and permission from [66], Copyright 2021, Nanoscale Research Letters). (**b**) Diagrams showing the construction, operation, and medicinal uses of electrochemical sensors based on nanomaterials. (Reprinted and permission from [68], Copyright 2021, Advanced NanoBiomed Research)

Moreover, hybrid nanomaterials facilitate the improvement of multifunctional biosensing systems. Incorporating chiral plasmonic hybrid nanostructures can beautify chiroptical homes, which are beneficial for sensing packages that require high sensitivity to molecular chirality [67]. Additionally, the use of nanomaterials in electrochemical sensors has been significantly reviewed, indicating their potential to beautify signal transduction mechanisms, thereby improving biosensors' overall sensitivity and response time [68]; using nanomaterials to construct, control, and electrochemical sensors for medicinal applications. See Fig. 7.4b.

The electrocatalytic properties of those substances, mainly in the context of glucose sensing, underscore their essential role in developing biosensing technology [69]. Furthermore, the utility of hybrid nanomaterials extends to biomedicine, where they are utilized for non-invasive diagnostics and healing programs. Hybrid nanomaterials have been employed in growing localized surface plasmon resonance (LSPR) biosensors, which leverage the electromagnetic fields around metallic nanoparticles to enhance detection limits for diverse biomolecules [70]. Functionalizing those nanomaterials with biomolecules, which includes aptamers or enzymes, similarly complements their specificity and sensitivity, making them suitable for a wide variety of biomedical programs [71].

7.6 Challenges and Opportunities

The integration of biosensors at the point-of-care (POC) with AI and bioinformatics is a major challenge, especially in terms of data management and diagnostic reliability. The complexity of the data generated by these biosensors requires advanced computational resources and robust frameworks, which are often lacking in resource-constrained environments [72, 73]. In addition, the performance of artificial intelligence models depends on the availability of high-quality, diverse datasets for training, which are often either limited or inconsistent in biosensor applications [74]. Studies emphasizing the dependence of diagnostic effects on the pleasant of input statistics display how this shortage can affect the accuracy and reliability of AI-assisted analysis [2, 74]. Furthermore, the powerful use of biosensors in clinical settings relies upon their improvement as portable, user-friendly and legally compliant devices [75, 76]. Solving these problems and growing the sensitivity and specificity of biosensors, in addition to their integration into allotted healthcare structures, relies upon the non-stop development of nanotechnology and system studying [77–80].

The widespread use of artificial intelligence and bioinformatics in the healthcare era is a good deal hampered by ethical and felony issues. Two major demanding situations are following rigorous privacy rules inclusive of GDPR and HIPAA and ensuring interoperability with existing healthcare systems [81]. The widespread use of artificial intelligence and bioinformatics in the Ethical questions about the usage of affected person records, including issues of consent and bias in synthetic intelligence models, complicates the regulatory process [82, 83]. Maintaining the high sensitivity and specificity of biosensors underneath diverse environmental and medical settings gives nonetheless any other technical problem [84]. Modern synthetic intelligence systems carried out to beautify sign processing, and error correction cannot completely offset the shortcomings of poorly tuned biosensor additives.

Another major obstacle is economics, especially related to implementation and production costs. Advanced materials and technologies are required for modern

POC-biosensor hybrid nanomaterials and AI-united Production Costs for platforms, which can limit access to low-resource environments [75, 85]. In addition, the absence of consistent methods for combining many biosensors, artificial intelligence systems and bioinformatics tools increases the challenge of reaching the correct interoperability, thus slowing down the speed of innovation and clinical translation [86–88].

Despite these difficulties, the ability to combine artificial intelligence and biography with POC biosensors continues to develop. Advanced machine learning and deep learning techniques, which analyze complex computer patterns and improve future modelling, provide a unique opportunity to improve clinical accuracy significantly. Clinical diagnosis is improved, and biosensors are more relevant to food safety and environmental monitoring [89, 90]. Especially in treating chronic diseases, the convergence of the portable biosensor with artificial intelligence and biochemistry promotes accurate-time health monitoring and individual medicine [91–93]. wearable technologies allow continuous physical data to be collected, which can offer action-provoking insights into unique health profiles when analyzed with artificial intelligence algorithms [94, 95].

Hybrid nanomaterials, such as graphene-based composites, improve point-of-care biosensor performance by improving sensitivity, endurance, and adaptation to different environments [96, 97]. This development makes it possible to develop reliable biosensors that can identify low-abundance biomarkers with extreme precision. Additionally, decentralized diagnostics are made possible by the scalability and portability of proof-of-concept biosensors in conjunction with cloud-based artificial intelligence systems; this aspect is particularly important during broad public health emergencies like pandemics [24, 90]. This centralized method improves real-time public health responses by hastening the general use of diagnostic tests.

The integration of point-of-care biosensors, smart devices and the Internet of Things will increase their application outdoors of conventional healthcare. This integrated gadget allows real-time tracking abilities in numerous utility areas, including health tracking, environmental monitoring, and food protection [98, 99]. Enhanced bioinformatics tools support global collaboration by permitting large-scale data sharing and reproducibility, accelerating the improvement and validation of new diagnostic technology [100]. Furthermore, regulatory help is developing as policymakers know more and more well known the transformative potential of AI-incorporated point-of-care biosensors in healthcare [101, 102]. This developing recognition is shaping a more supportive regulatory environment, fostering innovation and encouraging broader adoption.

The incorporation of point-of-care biosensors with artificial intelligence and bioinformatics has revolutionized diagnostic and health-tracking skills. The transformative ability of these technologies stays obvious, even in the face of ongoing challenges in records management, regulatory compliance, and cost, given the possibilities for innovation, increased accessibility, and superior healthcare effects.

7.7 Future Perspectives

The future of POC biosensors integrated with AI and bioinformatics is poised to redefine the landscape of diagnostics and customized remedies. As technological advancements boost up, next-era POC biosensors will inevitably characteristic unparalleled degrees of miniaturization, portability, and multifunctionality. These developments will be driven by breakthroughs in nanotechnology, which enable the creation of pretty sensitive and selective biosensors capable of detecting minute concentrations of biomarkers in complex biological matrices [103, 104]. Moreover, the integration of quantum computing with bioinformatics has the potential to revolutionize records evaluation, facilitating the rapid interpretation of complicated datasets generated with the aid of POC biosensors [105]. This capability is especially tremendous as the extent and complexity of data from next-generation sequencing (NGS) and different excessive-throughput technologies keep growing [106]. The synergy of that technology no longer best promises to beautify diagnostic accuracy but also to customize remedy strategies, therefore improving affected person effects and healthcare delivery [107].

An essential place of awareness may be the enhancement of actual-time monitoring and predictive abilities through superior ML algorithms. In addition to detecting anomalies, these algorithms will enable biosensors to predict disease progression and treatment outcomes [108, 109]. In the context of persistent illnesses, such predictive analytics could provide early intervention techniques tailored to the individual sufferer. Additionally, the improvement of adaptive AI structures that continuously research and enhance from new information inputs will similarly beautify the accuracy and reliability of diagnostic gear [110, 111].

POC biosensors powered by AI are another promising way to democratize healthcare. These devices could be used to provide superb diagnostics to underserved populations by reducing the need for centralized laboratories and specialized personnel [112]. In low-resource settings that lack traditional diagnostic infrastructure, this shift toward decentralized healthcare will have a particularly dramatic impact. It is possible to integrate POC biosensors seamlessly into virtual healthcare ecosystems, enabling real-time health assessments and remote consultations [113]. IoT and wearable technologies will enable POC biosensors to be used in more places beyond clinical settings. The incorporation of wearable biosensors in everyday accessories, such as clothing and watches, will enable individuals to monitor their health continuously [114, 115]. AI-driven analytics will enable these devices to deliver personalized insights and recommendations, paving the way for preventive medicine in the future [116, 117]. Furthermore, these technologies will be integrated with smart home systems and mobile applications, enabling users to be more engaged with therapeutic regimens and maintain compliance [118–120].

In addition to healthcare, POC biosensors incorporated with AI and bioinformatics will find elevated programs in environmental tracking, meal protection, and biodefense. Advanced biosensors capable of detecting contaminants, pathogens, and toxins with high specificity and sensitivity will play an important function in ensuring public safety and environmental sustainability [121, 122]. A robust reaction framework for rising challenges, including pandemics and bioterrorism, will be provided with the use of AI-driven analytics [16, 98]. To recognize those advancements, continued funding in interdisciplinary research and improvement can be essential. Collaborative efforts amongst scientists, engineers, clinicians, and policymakers will power innovation and address existing challenges, such as regulatory compliance and price reduction [123, 124]. The establishment of standardized protocols for integrating AI and bioinformatics with biosensors will, in addition, streamline the development and deployment of this technology, ensuring their reliability and scalability [125, 126]. The synergy between POC biosensors and synthetic intelligence and bioinformatics marks a revolution in diagnostics and health monitoring. Despite continuous challenges in data management, regulatory compliance, and value, these technologies nonetheless should transform strength based on the potential for innovation, greater accessibility, and better healthcare outcomes.

7.8 Conclusion

The convergence of biosensors, artificial intelligence (AI), and bioinformatics constitutes an enormous boost in diagnostic abilities. They offer unparalleled opportunities for customized medication, decentralized healthcare and actual-time fitness tracking. These technologies have established their potential to boost diagnostic accuracy, improve affected person consequences and extend entry to exceptional healthcare, especially in underserved and remote regions. Recent developments in system learning, nanotechnology, and bioinformatics have significantly improved the competencies of point-of-care biosensors, enabling them to serve as versatile tools for complex healthcare programs. Although extensive development has been made, impediments to tremendous adoption stay. Several obstacles impede the entire realization of those technologies, including integration, regulatory compliance, fee issues, and sensor optimization. Despite these demanding situations, even though it is being done with continuous multidisciplinary cooperation and investment in studies and improvement. Modern synthetic intelligence algorithms mixed with sturdy bioinformatics gear may want to help conquer present constraints and start the following technology of clever biosensors. The combined use of point-of-care biosensors, portable technologies, IoT systems and cloud-based platforms provides a transformation ability for diagnosis and health services. These advances will not only improve the efficiency of the healthcare system but will also promote better personal health management. In addition, the expansion of POC biosensor applications in areas such as environmental monitoring, food security, and bio-fence their versatility and broad social impact. In areas with diagnostics and the health care system, POC biosensors, with artificial intelligence and bioinformality, mark a paradigm shift. There is no doubt that these technologies can change global health with their development. They combine a new era with available, accurate and active treatment and provide creative answers to the nearest environment and medical problems.

References

1. Lim WY, Lan BL, Ramakrishnan N (2021) Emerging biosensors to detect severe acute respiratory syndrome coronavirus 2 (SARS-CoV-2): A review. Biosensors 11(11). https://doi.org/10.3390/bios11110434
2. Choi JR (2020) Development of Point-of-Care Biosensors for COVID-19. Front Chem 8. https://doi.org/10.3389/fchem.2020.00517
3. Herman R, Kravos NA, Jensterle M, Janež A, Dolžan V (2022) Metformin and insulin resistance: A review of the underlying mechanisms behind changes in GLUT4-mediated glucose transport. Int J Mol Sci 23(3). https://doi.org/10.3390/ijms23031264
4. Rasmi Y, Li X, Khan J, Ozer T, Choi JR (2021) Emerging point-of-care biosensors for rapid diagnosis of COVID-19: current progress, challenges, and future prospects. Anal Bioanal Chem 413(16):4137–4159. https://doi.org/10.1007/s00216-021-03377-6
5. Taha BA, Abbas EM, Kadhim AC, Azzahrani AS, Haider AJ, Chaudhary V, Arsad N (2024) Needle scattered light guided Chiplets-interfaced with AI for advanced biomedical application. Microelectron Eng 292:112228. https://doi.org/10.1016/j.mee.2024.112228
6. Taha BA, Addie AJ, Haider AJ, Kadhim AC, Azzahrani AS, Arsad N (2024) Needle-free targeted injections using bubble laser technology in therapeutics. Langmuir:1–12. https://doi.org/10.1021/acs.langmuir.4c03513
7. Chaudhary V, Taha BA, Lucky, Rustagi S, Khosla A, Papakonstantinou P, Bhalla N (2024) Nose-on-chip nanobiosensors for early detection of lung cancer breath biomarkers. ACS Sens. https://doi.org/10.1021/acssensors.4c01524
8. da Silva ETSG, Souto DEP, Barragan JTC, de F. Giarola J, de Moraes ACM, Kubota LT (2017) Electrochemical biosensors in point-of-care devices: recent advances and future trends. Chem Electro Chem 4(4):778–794. https://doi.org/10.1002/celc.201600758
9. Shumeiko V, Paltiel Y, Bisker G, Hayouka Z, Shoseyov O (2020) A paper-based near-infrared optical biosensor for quantitative detection of protease activity using peptide-encapsulated Swcnts. Sensors (Switzerland) 20(18):1–14. https://doi.org/10.3390/s20185247
10. Taha BA, Ahmed NM, Talreja RK, Haider AJ, Al Mashhadany Y, Al-Jubouri Q, Huddin AB, Mokhtar MHH, Rustagi S, Kaushik A, Chaudhary V, Arsad N (2024) Synergizing nanomaterials and artificial intelligence in advanced optical biosensors for precision antimicrobial resistance diagnosis. ACS Synth Biol. https://doi.org/10.1021/acssynbio.4c00070
11. Sun AC, Hall DA (2019) Point-of-care smartphone-based electrochemical biosensing. Electroanalysis 31(1):2–16. https://doi.org/10.1002/elan.201800474
12. Schary W, Paskali F, Rentschler S, Ruppert C, Wagner GE, Steinmetz I, Deigner HP, Kohl M (2022) Open-source, adaptable, all-in-one smartphone-based system for quantitative analysis of point-of-care diagnostics. Diagnostics 12(3):589. https://doi.org/10.3390/diagnostics12030589
13. Taha BA, Addie AJ, Kadhim AC, Azzahrani AS, Ahmed NM, Haider AJ, Chaudhary V, Arsad N (2024) Plasmonic-enabled nanostructures for designing the next generation of silicon photodetectors: trends, engineering and opportunities. Surf Interfaces 48:104334. https://doi.org/10.1016/j.surfin.2024.104334
14. Ahmed Taha B, Kadhim AC, Addie AJ, Haider AJ, Azzahrani AS, Raizada P, Rustagi S, Chaudhary V, Arsad N (2024) Advancing cancer diagnostics through multifaceted optical biosensors supported by nanomaterials and artificial intelligence: A panoramic outlook. Microchem J 205:111307. https://doi.org/10.1016/j.microc.2024.111307
15. Baluta S, Cabaj J, Malecha K (2020) Biosensors technologies for point-of-care testing—a review. Periodica polytechnica Electrical engineering and computer science 64(4):325–333. https://doi.org/10.3311/PPee.15358
16. Omidfar K, Ahmadi A, Syedmoradi L, Khoshfetrat SM, Larijani B (2020) Point-of-care biosensors in medicine: A brief overview of our achievements in this field based on the conducted research in EMRI (endocrinology and metabolism research Institute of Tehran University of

Medical Sciences) over the past fourteen years. J Diabetes Metab Disord:1455–1459. https://doi.org/10.1007/s40200-020-00668-0
17. Nishitani S, Man Y, Noguchi T, Sakata T (2022) Polyaniline-based nanostructure Interface for signal-to-noise ratio enhancement in potentiometric enzyme-free biosensors. Adv Mater Interfaces 9(27):2201029. https://doi.org/10.1002/admi.202201029
18. Inan H, Poyraz M, Inci F, Lifson MA, Baday M, Cunningham BT, Demirci U (2017) Photonic crystals: emerging biosensors and their promise for point-of-care applications. Chem Soc Rev 46(2):366–388. https://doi.org/10.1039/c6cs00206d
19. Cui F, Yue Y, Zhang Y, Zhang Z, Zhou HS (2020) Advancing biosensors with machine learning. ACS Sens 5(11):3346–3364. https://doi.org/10.1021/acssensors.0c01424
20. Taha BA, Al Mashhadany Y, Al-Jubouri Q, Haider AJ, Chaudhary V, Apsari R, Arsad N (2023) Uncovering the morphological differences between SARS-CoV-2 and SARS-CoV based on transmission electron microscopy images. Microbes Infect:105187. https://doi.org/10.1016/j.micinf.2023.105187
21. Taha BA, Al Mashhadany Y, Al-Jumaily AHJ, Zan MSDB, Arsad N (2022) SARS-CoV-2 morphometry analysis and prediction of real virus levels based on full recurrent neural network using TEM images. Viruses, Multidisciplinary Digital Publishing Institute 14(11):2386
22. Tahaa BA, Yeha RMM, Sapiee NM, Al Mashhadany Y, Haider AJ, M. H. H. M. & N. A (2024) Superpixel segmentation-enabled transmission electron microscopy images for rapid and accurate detection of coronavirus. J Kejuruteraan 36(3). https://doi.org/10.17576/jkukm-2024-36(3)-16. Superpixel
23. Giordano GF, Ferreira LF, Bezerra ÍRS, Barbosa JA, Costa JNY, Pimentel GJC, Lima RS (2023) Machine learning toward high-performance electrochemical sensors. Anal Bioanal Chem 415(18):3683–3692. https://doi.org/10.1007/s00216-023-04514-z
24. Qureshi R, Irfan M, Ali H, Khan A, Nittala AS, Ali S, Shah A, Gondal TM, Sadak F, Shah Z, Hadi MU, Khan S, Al-Tashi Q, Wu J, Bermak A, Alam T (2023) Artificial intelligence and biosensors in healthcare and its clinical relevance: a review. IEEE Access 11:61600–61620. https://doi.org/10.1109/ACCESS.2023.3285596
25. Beabout K, Bernhards CB, Thakur M, Turner KB, Cole SD, Walper SA, Chávez JL, Lux MW (2021) Optimization of heavy metal sensors based on transcription factors and cell-free expression systems. ACS Synth Biol 10(11):3040–3054. https://doi.org/10.1021/acssynbio.1c00331
26. Chen J, Vishweshwaraiah YL, Mailman RB, Tabdanov ED, Dokholyan NV (2023) A non-commutative combinatorial protein logic circuit controls cell orientation in nanoenvironments. Sci Adv 9(21):1–14. https://doi.org/10.1126/sciadv.adg1062
27. Kim H, Lee W, Yoon Y (2019) Heavy metal(loid) biosensor based on Split-enhanced green fluorescent protein: development and characterization. Appl Microbiol Biotechnol 103(15):6345–6352. https://doi.org/10.1007/s00253-019-09908-7
28. Mahmud MS, Fang H, Wang H, Carreiro S, Boyer E, Automatic Detection of Opioid Intake Using Wearable Biosensor (2018) International Conference on Computing. ICNC 2018(2018):784–788. https://doi.org/10.1109/ICCNC.2018.8390334
29. Mazuryk J, Klepacka K, Kutner W, Sharma PS (2023) Glyphosate separating and sensing for precision agriculture and environmental protection in the era of smart materials. Environ Sci Technol 57(27):9898–9924. https://doi.org/10.1021/acs.est.3c01269
30. Giwa AS, Maurice NJ, Ali N (2023) Construction of a novel oxalic acid biosensor based on the combination of tissue enzyme and peroxide mimic enzyme. PRO 11(10). https://doi.org/10.3390/pr11103012
31. Bazhenov S, Novoyatlova U, Scheglova E, Fomin V, Khrulnova S, Melkina O, Chistyakov V, Manukhov I (2021) Influence of the Luxr regulatory gene dosage and expression level on the sensitivity of the whole-cell biosensor to acyl-Homoserine lactone. Biosensors 11(6). https://doi.org/10.3390/bios11060166
32. Taha BA, Al Mashhadany Y, Mokhtar MHH, Zan MSDB, Arsad N (2020) An analysis review of detection coronavirus disease 2019 (Covid-19) based on biosensor application. Sensors (Switzerland) 20(23):1–29. https://doi.org/10.3390/s20236764

33. Khosravi Ardakani H, Gerami M, Chashmpoosh M, Omidifar N, Gholami A (2022) Recent progress in nanobiosensors for precise detection of blood glucose level. Biochem Res Int 2022. https://doi.org/10.1155/2022/2964705
34. Rong G, Corrie SR, Clark HA (2017) In vivo biosensing: progress and perspectives. ACS Sens 2(3):327–338. https://doi.org/10.1021/acssensors.6b00834
35. Tuoheti A, Aiassa S, Criscuolo F, Stradolini F, Tzouvadaki I, Carrara S, Demarchi D (2020) New approach for making standard the development of biosensing devices by a modular multi-purpose design. IEEE Trans Nanobioscience 19(3):339–346. https://doi.org/10.1109/TNB.2020.2995230
36. Suva M, Bhatia G (2024) Artificial intelligence in addiction: challenges and opportunities. Indian J Psychol Med. https://doi.org/10.1177/02537176241274148
37. Verma AK, Noumani A, Yadav AK, Solanki PR (2023) FRET based biosensor: principle applications recent advances and challenges. Diagnostics 13(8). https://doi.org/10.3390/diagnostics13081375
38. Madhu M, Santhoshkumar S, Tseng W-B, Tseng W-L (2023) Maximizing analytical precision: exploring the advantages of Ratiometric strategy in fluorescence, Raman, electrochemical, and mass spectrometry detection. Front Analytic Sci 3:1–14. https://doi.org/10.3389/frans.2023.1258558
39. Taha BA, Al-Tahar IA, Addie AJ, Mahdi AB, Haider AJ, Al Mashhadany Y, Chaudhary V, Arsad N (2024) Nanophotonic catheters: a lens into the body for biosensing and biomedical imaging. Applied Mater Today 38:102229. https://doi.org/10.1016/j.apmt.2024.102229
40. Ahmed Taha B, Addie AJ, Saeed AQ, Haider AJ, Chaudhary V, Arsad N (2024) Nanostructured photonics probes: A transformative approach in neurotherapeutics and brain circuitry. Neuroscience 562:106–124. https://doi.org/10.1016/j.neuroscience.2024.10.046
41. Kadhim, A. C., Azzahrani, A. S., Taha, B. A. Quantitative analysis of three-dimensional refractive index distribution in a biological volume sample for biomedical applications. 2024
42. Taha BA, Addie AJ, Abbas EM, Aubaidan BH, Ahmed NM, Haider AJ, Chaudhary V, Arsad N (2024) Biophotonics and nanorobotics for biomedical imaging, biosensing, drug delivery, and therapy. J Photochem Photobiol C: Photochem Rev 60–61:100678. https://doi.org/10.1016/j.jphotochemrev.2024.100678
43. Tokpah DP, IŞIN A, Erkurt H (2021) Assessment of facile biosensors for rapid detection of coronavirus a review for designing real-time monitoring systems. Int J Front Biol Pharm Res 1(2):036–041. https://doi.org/10.53294/ijfbpr.2021.1.2.0051
44. Zhang L, Yang Q, Zhu Z (2024) The application of multi-parameter multi-modal technology integrating biological sensors and artificial intelligence in the rapid detection of food contaminants. Foods 13(12). https://doi.org/10.3390/foods13121936
45. Jin S, Lednev IK, Jung YM (2024) Recent trends in surface-enhanced Raman spectroscopy-based biosensors: label-free early disease diagnosis. J Phys Chem C 128(22):8861–8873. https://doi.org/10.1021/acs.jpcc.4c02011
46. Lu N, Chen J, Rao Z, Guo B, Xu Y (2023) Recent advances of biosensors for detection of multiple antibiotics. Biosensors 13(9). https://doi.org/10.3390/bios13090850
47. Fu W, Yu B, Ji D, Zhou Z, Li X, Wang R, Lu W, Sun Y, Dai Y (2024) Intelligent fibers and textiles for wearable biosensors. Responsive Materials. https://doi.org/10.1002/rpm.20240018
48. Jin X, Cai A, Xu T, Zhang X (2023) Artificial intelligence biosensors for continuous glucose monitoring. Interdiscip Mater 2(2):290–307. https://doi.org/10.1002/idm2.12069
49. Li L, Tu R, Song G, Cheng J, Chen W, Li L, Wang L, Wang Q (2019) Development of a synthetic 3-dehydroshikimate biosensor in Escherichia Coli for metabolite monitoring and genetic screening. ACS Synth Biol 8(2):297–306. https://doi.org/10.1021/acssynbio.8b00317
50. Zhang L, Guo W, Lu Y (2020) Advances in cell-free biosensors: principle, mechanism, and applications. Biotechnol J 15(9):1–14. https://doi.org/10.1002/biot.202000187
51. Nasirahmadi S, Zargan J (2020) Research paper: bioinformatics analysis of linear B-cell Viscumin toxin epitope with potential use in molecularly imprinted polymer biosensors. Int J Med Toxicol Forensic Med 10(1):1–8. https://doi.org/10.32598/ijmtfm.v10i1.26172

52. Shukla N, Srivastava N, Gupta R, Srivastava P, Narayan J (2023) COVID variants, villain and victory: a bioinformatics perspective. Microorganisms 11(8). https://doi.org/10.3390/microorganisms11082039
53. Georgeson P, Syme A, Sloggett C, Chung J, Dashnow H, Milton M, Lonsdale A, Powell D, Seemann T, Pope B (2019) Bionitio: demonstrating and facilitating best practices for bioinformatics command-line software. GigaScience 8(9):1–10. https://doi.org/10.1093/gigascience/giz109
54. Fatima A, Younas I, Ali MW (2022) An overview on recent advances in biosensor technology and its future application. Arch Pharm Pract 13(1):5–10. https://doi.org/10.51847/LToGI43jil
55. Tomichan R, Sharma A, Akash K, Siddiqui AA, Dubey A, Upadhyay TK, Kumar D, Pandey S, Nagraik R (2023) Insight of smart biosensors for COVID-19: a review. Luminescence 38(7):1102–1110. https://doi.org/10.1002/bio.4430
56. Cook CE, Lopez R, Stroe O, Cochrane G, Brooksbank C, Birney E, Apweiler R (2019) The European bioinformatics Institute in 2018: tools, infrastructure and training. Nucleic Acids Res 47(D1):D15–D22. https://doi.org/10.1093/nar/gky1124
57. Kamoun C, Roméjon J, de Soyres H, Gallois A, Girard E, Hupé P (2021) Biogitflow: Development Workflow Protocols for Bioinformatics Pipelines with Git and GitLab [Version 2; Peer Review: 1 Approved, 1 Approved with Reservations]. F1000Research 9:1–19. https://doi.org/10.12688/F1000RESEARCH.24714.2
58. Anashkina AA, Leberfarb EY, Orlov YL (2021) Recent trends in cancer genomics and bioinformatics tools development. Int J Mol Sci 22(22). https://doi.org/10.3390/ijms222212146
59. Pham C, Stogios PJ, Savchenko A, Mahadevan R (2024) Design and characterization of a generalist biosensor for indole derivatives. ACS Synth Biol 13(7):2246–2252. https://doi.org/10.1021/acssynbio.3c00736
60. Curulli A (2023) Functional nanomaterials enhancing electrochemical biosensors as smart tools for detecting infectious viral diseases. Molecules 28(9):3777. https://doi.org/10.3390/molecules28093777
61. Zandi M, Zandi S, Mohammadi R, Hosseini P, Teymouri S, Soltani S, Rasouli A (2022) Biosensor as an alternative diagnostic method for rabies virus detection: A literature review. Biotechnol Appl Biochem 69(4):1348–1353. https://doi.org/10.1002/bab.2207
62. Taha BA, Abdulrahm ZM, Addie AJ, Haider AJ, Alkawaz AN, Yaqoob IAM, Arsad N (2025) Advancing optical nanosensors with artificial intelligence: A powerful tool to identify disease-specific biomarkers in multi-omics profiling. Talanta 287(January):127693. https://doi.org/10.1016/j.talanta.2025.127693
63. Taha BA, Addie AJ, Haider AJ, Norhana A (2025) Nanosensors based on breathomics for human disease diagnosis: a new frontier in personalized healthcare. Bio Nano Sci. https://doi.org/10.1007/s12668-025-01876-9
64. Foroutan B, Abbasian Najafabadi AR (2021) Capabilities of bioinformatics tools for optimizing physicochemical features of proteins used in nano biosensors: A short overview of the tools related to bioinformatics. Biochem Biophys Rep 27:101094. https://doi.org/10.1016/j.bbrep.2021.101094
65. Kwon EH, Kim M, Lee CY, Kim M, Park YD (2022) Metal-organic-framework-decorated carbon nanofibers with enhanced gas sensitivity when incorporated into an organic semiconductor-based gas sensor. ACS Appl Mater Interfaces 14(8):10637–10647. https://doi.org/10.1021/acsami.1c24740
66. Aykaç A, Gergeroglu H, Beşli B, Akkaş EÖ, Yavaş A, Güler S, Güneş F, Erol M (2021) An overview on recent progress of metal oxide/graphene/CNTs-based nanobiosensors. Nanoscale Res Letter 16(1). https://doi.org/10.1186/s11671-021-03519-w
67. Tan L, Fu W, Gao Q, Wang P p (2024) Chiral Plasmonic hybrid nanostructures: a gateway to advanced Chiroptical materials. Adv Mater 36(3):2309033. https://doi.org/10.1002/adma.202309033
68. Liu X, Huang L, Qian K (2021) Nanomaterial-based electrochemical sensors: mechanism, preparation, and application in biomedicine. Adv Nano Biomed Res 1(6). https://doi.org/10.1002/anbr.202000104

69. Thatikayala D, Ponnamma D, Sadasivuni KK, Cabibihan JJ, Al-Ali AK, Malik RA, Min B (2020) Progress of advanced nanomaterials in the non-enzymatic electrochemical sensing of glucose and H2O2. Biosensors 10(11). https://doi.org/10.3390/BIOS10110151
70. Li M, Singh R, Wang Y, Marques C, Zhang B, Kumar S (2022) Advances in novel nanomaterial-based optical fiber biosensors—a review. Biosensors 12(10). https://doi.org/10.3390/bios12100843
71. Vázquez-gonzález M, Willner I (2021) Aptamer-functionalized hybrid nanostructures for sensing, drug delivery, catalysis and mechanical applications. Int J Mol Sci 22(4):1–32. https://doi.org/10.3390/ijms22041803
72. Bhalla N, Pan Y, Yang Z, Payam AF (2020) Opportunities and challenges for biosensors and nanoscale analytical tools for pandemics: COVID-19. ACS Nano 14(7):7783–7807. https://doi.org/10.1021/acsnano.0c04421
73. Harito C, Khalil M, Septiani NLW, Dewi KK, Hardiansyah A, Yuliarto B, Walsh FC (2022) Trends in nanomaterial-based biosensors for viral detection. Nano Futures 6(2):22005. https://doi.org/10.1088/2399-1984/ac701d
74. Harada Y, Katsukura S, Kawamura R, Shimizu T (2021) Efficacy of artificial-intelligence-driven differential-diagnosis list on the diagnostic accuracy of physicians: an open-label randomized controlled study. Int J Environ Res Public Health 18(4):1–10. https://doi.org/10.3390/ijerph18042086
75. Jin J, Guo J, Guo J, Li D (2024) Carbon-Based Biosensor in Point of Care Setting. Adv Sensor Res 3(10). https://doi.org/10.1002/adsr.202400037
76. Pohanka M (2022) Progress in biosensors for the point-of-care diagnosis of COVID-19. Sensors 22(19):7423. https://doi.org/10.3390/s22197423
77. Manoharan Nair Sudha Kumari S, Thankappan Suryabai X (2024) Sensing the future—frontiers in biosensors: exploring classifications, principles, and recent advances. ACS Omega 9(50):48918–48987. https://doi.org/10.1021/acsomega.4c07991
78. Kumar S, Sharma R, Bhawna, Gupta A, Singh P, Kalia S, Thakur P, Kumar V (2022) Prospects of biosensors based on functionalized and nanostructured solitary materials: detection of viral infections and other risks. ACS Omega 7(26):22073–22088. https://doi.org/10.1021/acsomega.2c01033
79. Taha BA, Abdulateef SA, Addie AJ, Muneam SA, Muneam NA, Haider AJ, Ahmed NM, Chaudhary V, Arsad N (2025) Paradigm of nanophotonics integrated smart contact lenses: a new frontier in wearable healthcare. Mater Res Bull 190:113511. https://doi.org/10.1016/j.materresbull.2025.113511
80. Taha BA, Addie AJ, Chahal S, Haider AJ, Rustagi S, Arsad N, Chaudhary V (2024) Unlocking new frontiers in healthcare: the impact of nano-optical biosensors on personalized medical diagnostics. J Biotechnol 400:29–47. https://doi.org/10.1016/j.jbiotec.2025.02.005
81. Mohammad Amini M, Jesus M, Fanaei Sheikholeslami D, Alves P, Hassanzadeh Benam A, Hariri F (2023) Artificial intelligence ethics and challenges in healthcare applications: a comprehensive review in the context of the European GDPR mandate. Machine Learning and Knowledge Extraction 5(3):1023–1035. https://doi.org/10.3390/make5030053
82. Hoseini M (2023) Patient experiences with AI in healthcare settings. AI and Tech in Behavioral and Social Sciences 1(3):12–18. https://doi.org/10.61838/kman.aitech.1.3.3
83. Harishbhai Tilala M, Kumar Chenchala P, Choppadandi A, Kaur J, Naguri S, Saoji R, Devaguptapu B (2024) Ethical considerations in the use of artificial intelligence and machine learning in health care: A comprehensive review. Cureus. https://doi.org/10.7759/cureus.62443
84. Ley B, Satyagraha AW, Kibria MG, Armstrong J, Bancone G, Bei AK, Bizilj G, Brito M, Ding XC, Domingo GJ, von Fricken ME, Gornsawun G, Lam B, Menard D, Monteiro W, Ongarello S, Pal S, Panggalo LV, Parikh S, Pfeffer DA, Price RN, da Silva Orfano A, Wade M, Wojnarski M, Worachet K, Yar A, Alam MS, Howes RE (2022) Repeatability and reproducibility of a handheld quantitative G6PD diagnostic. PLoS Negl Trop Dis 16(2):e0010174. https://doi.org/10.1371/journal.pntd.0010174

85. Aslan Y, Atabay M, Chowdhury HK, Göktürk I, Saylan Y, Inci F (2023) Aptamer-based point-of-care devices: emerging technologies and integration of computational methods. Biosensors 13(5):569. https://doi.org/10.3390/bios13050569
86. Kuupiel D, Bawontuo V, Drain PK, Gwala N, Mashamba-Thompson TP (2019) Supply chain management and accessibility to point-of-care testing in resource-limited settings: a systematic scoping review. BMC Health Serv Res 19(1):519. https://doi.org/10.1186/s12913-019-4351-3
87. Maluleke K, Musekiwa A, Kgarosi K, Gregor EM, Dlangalala T, Nkambule S, Mashamba-Thompson T (2021) A scoping review of supply chain Management Systems for Point of care diagnostic services: Optimising Covid-19 testing capacity in resource-limited settings. Diagnostics 11(12):2299. https://doi.org/10.3390/diagnostics11122299
88. Taha BA, Al-Rawi MA, Addie AJ, Abdulateef SA, Haider AJ, Chaudhary V, Arsad N (2025) Nanomaterial-enhanced biosensors for polycystic ovarian syndrome diagnosis and pathophysiological insights. Microchim Acta 192(8):547. https://doi.org/10.1007/s00604-025-07415-3
89. Huang JD, Wang J, Ramsey E, Leavey G, Chico TJA, Condell J (2022) Applying artificial intelligence to wearable sensor data to diagnose and predict cardiovascular disease: A review. Sensors 22(20):8002. https://doi.org/10.3390/s22208002
90. Flynn CD, Chang D (2024) Artificial intelligence in point-of-care biosensing: challenges and opportunities. Diagnostics 14(11):1100. https://doi.org/10.3390/diagnostics14111100
91. Secara I-A, Hordiiuk D (2024) Personalized health monitoring systems: integrating wearable and AI. J Intell Learn Syst Appl 16(02):44–52. https://doi.org/10.4236/jilsa.2024.162004
92. Shajari S, Kuruvinashetti K, Komeili A, Sundararaj U (2023) The emergence of AI-based wearable sensors for digital health technology: a review. Sensors 23(23):9498. https://doi.org/10.3390/s23239498
93. Taha BA, Sulaiman GM, Addie AJ, Khalil KAA, Ahmed EM, Chaudhary V, Arsad N (2025) Multifunctional Nanophotonic photoacoustic biosensors: a new era in molecular imaging—guided deep-tissue cancer monitoring. Methods 242(June):1–23. https://doi.org/10.1016/j.ymeth.2025.06.005
94. Xian X (2023) Frontiers of wearable biosensors for human health monitoring. Biosensors 13(11):964. https://doi.org/10.3390/bios13110964
95. Neri L, Oberdier MT, van Abeelen KCJ, Menghini L, Tumarkin E, Tripathi H, Jaipalli S, Orro A, Paolocci N, Gallelli I, Dall'Olio M, Beker A, Carrick RT, Borghi C, Halperin HR (2023) Electrocardiogram monitoring wearable devices and artificial-intelligence-enabled diagnostic capabilities: a review. *Sensors* 23(10):4805. https://doi.org/10.3390/s23104805
96. Gao J, Gao Y, Han Y, Pang J, Wang C, Wang Y, Liu H, Zhang Y, Han L (2020) Ultrasensitive label-free MiRNA sensing based on a flexible graphene field-effect transistor without functionalization. ACS Appl Electronic Mater 2(4):1090–1098. https://doi.org/10.1021/acsaelm.0c00095
97. Irkham I, Ibrahim AU, Pwavodi PC, Al-Turjman F, Hartati YW (2023) Smart graphene-based electrochemical nanobiosensor for clinical diagnosis: review. Sensors 23(4):1–27. https://doi.org/10.3390/s23042240
98. Parihar A, Yadav S, Sadique MA, Ranjan P, Kumar N, Singhal A, Khare V, Khan R, Natarajan S, Srivastava AK (2023) Internet-of-medical-things integrated point-of-care biosensing devices for infectious diseases: toward better preparedness for futuristic pandemics. Bioengin Transl Med 8(3). https://doi.org/10.1002/btm2.10481
99. Choi JR, Yong KW, Choi JY, Cowie AC (2019) Emerging point-of-care technologies for food safety analysis. Sensors 19(4):817. https://doi.org/10.3390/s19040817
100. Lorenzo-Villegas DL, Gohil NV, Lamo P, Gurajala S, Bagiu IC, Vulcanescu DD, Horhat FG, Sorop VB, Diaconu M, Sorop MI, Oprisoni A, Horhat RM, Susan M, Mohana Sundaram AS (2023) Innovative biosensing approaches for swift identification of candida species, intrusive pathogenic organisms. Life 13(10):2099. https://doi.org/10.3390/life13102099
101. Stevenson H, Radha Shanmugam N, Paneer Selvam A, Prasad S (2018) The anatomy of a nonfaradaic electrochemical biosensor. SLAS Technol 23(1):5–15. https://doi.org/10.1177/2472630317738700

102. Sánchez-Salcedo R, Sharma P, Voelcker NH (2025) Advancements in porous silicon biosensors for point of care, wearable, and implantable applications. ACS Appl Mater Interfaces 17(2):2814–2843. https://doi.org/10.1021/acsami.4c18273
103. Fan M, Weng Y, Liu Y, Lu Y, Xu L, Ye J, Lin D, Qiu S, Feng S (2024) Surface-enhanced raman spectroscopy-based optical biosensor for liquid biopsy: toward precision medicine. Laser and Photonics Rev 18(5). https://doi.org/10.1002/lpor.202301072
104. Khan AH, Noordin R (2020) Serological and molecular rapid diagnostic tests for toxoplasma infection in humans and animals. Eur J Clin Microbiol Infect Dis 39(1):19–30. https://doi.org/10.1007/s10096-019-03680-2
105. Das B, Franco JL, Logan N, Balasubramanian P, Kim MI, Cao C (2021) Nanozymes in point-of-care diagnosis: an emerging futuristic approach for biosensing. Nano-Micro Letter 13(1). https://doi.org/10.1007/s40820-021-00717-0
106. Gullapalli RR (2020) Evaluation of commercial next-generation sequencing bioinformatics software solutions. J Mol Diagn 22(2):147–158. https://doi.org/10.1016/j.jmoldx.2019.09.007
107. Sun H, Peng G, Chen K, Xiong Z, Zhuang Y, Liu M, Ning X, Yang H, Deng J (2023) Identification of EGFR as an essential regulator in chondrocytes ferroptosis of osteoarthritis using bioinformatics, in vivo, and in vitro study. Heliyon 9(9):e19975. https://doi.org/10.1016/j.heliyon.2023.e19975
108. Ansari MA, Verma D, Hamizan MA, Mukherjee MD, Mohd-Naim NF, Ahmed MU (2025) Trends in Aptasensing and the enhancement of diagnostic efficiency and accuracy. ACS Synth Biol 14(1):21–40. https://doi.org/10.1021/acssynbio.4c00591
109. Vashistha R, Dangi AK, Kumar A, Chhabra D, Shukla P (2018) Futuristic biosensors for cardiac health care: an artificial intelligence approach. 3 Biotech 8(8). https://doi.org/10.1007/s13205-018-1368-y
110. Wang Y, Wagner AD, Liu S, Kingwara L, Oyaro P, Brown E, Karauki E, Yongo N, Bowen N, Kiiru J, Hassan S, Patel R (2024) Using queueing models as a decision support tool in allocating point-of-care HIV viral load testing machines in Kisumu County, Kenya. Health Policy Plan 39(1):44–55. https://doi.org/10.1093/heapol/czad111
111. Pabitha C, Kalpana V, Sonia ESV, Pushpalatha A, Mahendran G, Sivarajan S (2023) Development and implementation of an intelligent health monitoring system using IoT and advanced machine learning techniques. J Mach Comput 3(4):456–464. https://doi.org/10.53759/7669/jmc202303037
112. Aylward BS, Abbas H, Taraman S, Salomon C, Gal-Szabo D, Kraft C, Ehwerhemuepha L, Chang A, Wall DP (2023) An introduction to artificial intelligence in developmental and behavioral pediatrics. J Dev Behav Pediatr 44(2):E126–E134. https://doi.org/10.1097/DBP.0000000000001149
113. Crigger E, Reinbold K, Hanson C, Kao A, Blake K, Irons M (2022) Trustworthy augmented intelligence in health care. J Med Syst 46(2). https://doi.org/10.1007/s10916-021-01790-z
114. Ji W, Zhu J, Wu W, Wang N, Wang J, Wu J, Wu Q, Wang X, Yu C, Wei G, Li L, Huo F (2021) Wearable sweat biosensors refresh personalized health/medical diagnostics. Research 2021. https://doi.org/10.34133/2021/9757126
115. Kim J, Campbell AS, de Ávila BEF, Wang J (2019) Wearable biosensors for healthcare monitoring. Nat Biotechnol 37(4):389–406. https://doi.org/10.1038/s41587-019-0045-y
116. Bandodkar AJ, Jeang WJ, Ghaffari R, Rogers JA (2019) Wearable sensors for biochemical sweat analysis. Annu Rev Anal Chem 12(1):1–22. https://doi.org/10.1146/annurev-anchem-061318-114910
117. Zhang K, Wang J, Liu T, Luo Y, Loh XJ, Chen X (2021) Machine Learning-Reinforced Noninvasive Biosensors for Healthcare. Adv Healthcare Mater 10(17). https://doi.org/10.1002/adhm.202100734
118. Zheng Y, Omar R, Zhang R, Tang N, Khatib M, Xu Q, Milyutin Y, Saliba W, Broza YY, Wu W, Yuan M, Haick H (2022) A wearable microneedle-based extended gate transistor for real-time detection of sodium in interstitial fluids. Adv Mater 34(10). https://doi.org/10.1002/adma.202108607

119. Psoma SD, Kanthou C (2023) Wearable insulin biosensors for diabetes management: advances and challenges. Biosensors 13(7):719. https://doi.org/10.3390/bios13070719
120. Qiao L, Benzigar MR, Subramony JA, Lovell NH, Liu G (2020) Advances in sweat wearables: sample extraction, real-time biosensing, and flexible platforms. ACS Appl Mater Interfaces 12(30):34337–34361. https://doi.org/10.1021/acsami.0c07614
121. Cesewski E, Johnson BN (2020) Electrochemical biosensors for pathogen detection. Biosens Bioelectron 159:112214. https://doi.org/10.1016/j.bios.2020.112214
122. Russo MJ, Han M, Desroches PE, Manasa CS, Dennaoui J, Quigley AF, Kapsa RMI, Moulton SE, Guijt RM, Greene GW, Silva SM (2021) Antifouling strategies for electrochemical biosensing: mechanisms and performance toward point of care based diagnostic applications. ACS Sens 6(4):1482–1507. https://doi.org/10.1021/acssensors.1c00390
123. Kim D, Min J, Ko SH (2024) Recent Developments and Future Directions of Wearable Skin Biosignal Sensors. Adv Sensor Res 3(2). https://doi.org/10.1002/adsr.202300118
124. Sam MFM, Ismail AFMF, Bakar KA, Ahamat A, Qureshi MI (2022) The effectiveness of IoT based wearable devices and potential cybersecurity risks: A systematic literature review from the last decade. Int J Online Biomed Eng 18(9):56–73. https://doi.org/10.3991/ijoe.v18i09.32255
125. Ferreira JJ, Fernandes CI, Rammal HG, Veiga PM (2021) Wearable technology and consumer interaction: a systematic review and research agenda. Comput Hum Behav 118:106710. https://doi.org/10.1016/j.chb.2021.106710
126. Ngayua EN (2021) Integration of smart wearable devices and cloud computing in the Kenyan public health care system. Inform Knowl Manag. https://doi.org/10.7176/IKM/11-4-04

8 Biosensors into Surveillance Systems

Sarvesh B. Jadhav, Sadaf Shaikh, Sumedh Yewale, Aagam L. Bamb, Vedashree Sirdeshmukh, and Chandrakant Tagad

8.1 Introduction

Antimicrobial resistance (AMR) is a natural phenomenon that is accelerated by the misuse and overuse of antibiotics in the fields of agriculture, veterinary medicine, and human health. It results in the survival of resistant strains, making treatments ineffective thereby increasing mortality, prolonged hospital stays, and higher healthcare costs [1–3].

Decades of advancement in contemporary medicine are at risk due to the emergence of AMR, which has emerged as a serious public health concern [4–6]. It jeopardizes the management of infectious disorders and compromises medical procedures where infection control is essential, such as organ transplants, chemotherapy, and operations.

All authors have equally contributed to this chapter.

S. B. Jadhav
SoilSens Pvt. Ltd., Pune, India

S. Shaikh
Syngene International Limited, Hyderabad, India

S. Yewale
University of Michigan, Ann Arbor, MI, USA

A. L. Bamb
Biochemical Science Division, National Chemical Laboratory, Pune, India

V. Sirdeshmukh (✉)
Defence Institute of Advanced Technology, Pune, India

C. Tagad (✉)
Department of Biochemistry, SBES College, S.B.E.S. College of Science, Chhatrapati Sambhajinagar (Aurangabad), Maharashtra, India

V. Chaudhary, N. Bhalla (eds.), *Biosensors for Tackling Antimicrobial Resistance (AMR)*, https://doi.org/10.1007/978-981-95-9151-0_8

AMR surveillance is crucial to track developments in resistance, stop outbreaks, and direct the formulation of antibiotic stewardship policies. Surveillance systems are the backbone of efforts to mitigate AMR. They enable real-time detection of resistance trends and hotspots, helping public health authorities implement timely interventions. Despite their effectiveness, conventional techniques like culture and sensitivity testing are time-consuming, labour-intensive, and resource-intensive [7, 8]. These drawbacks render them inappropriate for quick, extensive monitoring. Therefore, it is necessary to integrate cutting-edge technologies like biosensors that can deliver data more quickly, accurately, and economically.

Biosensors are analytical tools that detect biological molecules and convert their presence or interaction into measurable signals [9–11]. There are three primary components that make up these devices: a biological recognition element (such as antibodies, enzymes, DNA, RNA, and cells) that is connected to a substrate (such as silicon, gold, glass, and polymers), and a transducer that generates a signal to convert the interaction with the target into a signal that can be measured and quantified with greater ease.

As per mentioned in Fig. 8.1 a signal (such as fluorescence, heat generation, colour changes, oscillatory frequency, or conductivity) is produced by the chemical reaction and converted into a measurable indicator that is directly proportional to the signal's magnitude [12].

In AMR surveillance, biosensors are uniquely suited to detect: Antibiotic residues in water, soil, and food, resistance genes in environmental or clinical samples, and biomarkers of microbial activity, signalling the presence of resistant pathogens. Their versatility, portability, and ability to integrate with digital technologies such as IoT make them indispensable in building next-generation AMR monitoring systems.

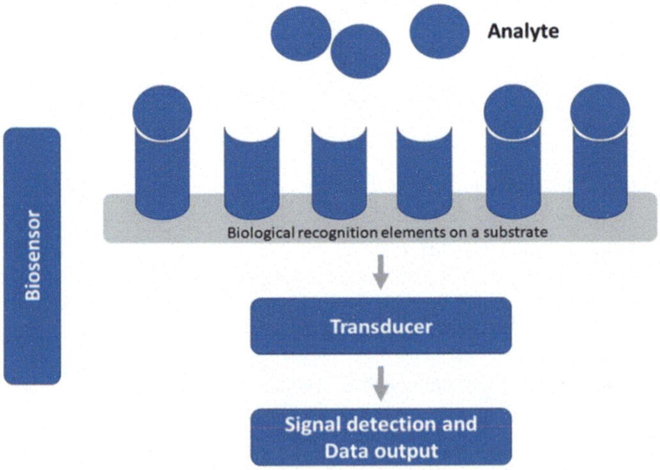

Fig. 8.1 General characteristics and components of a biosensor [12]

8.1.1 Objectives and Scope of the Chapter

Integrating biosensors into surveillance systems represents a transformative approach to combatting antimicrobial resistance. Conventional methods can take over 24 h to yield results, while biosensors can provide rapid diagnostics within hours or even minutes. This rapid turnaround is necessary for making therapeutic decisions in a timely manner and for providing effective therapy for infections that are caused by organisms that are resistant to treatment [13]. By providing rapid, sensitive, and cost-effective detection methods, biosensors can significantly enhance our ability to monitor AMR in clinical and environmental contexts, ultimately improving patient outcomes and public health strategies.

8.2 Overview of Biosensor Technologies for Surveillance

8.2.1 Types of Biosensors

Advancements in biosensor technology have broadened their applications in public health and beyond. This section provides a detailed examination of the types of biosensors, their key components, and recent innovations enhancing their utility in AMR surveillance.

8.2.1.1 Electrochemical Biosensors

Electrochemical biosensors are among the most widely used in AMR surveillance. They detect changes in electrical properties, such as current or voltage, resulting from biological interactions [14]. These sensors are beneficial for quantifying antibiotics and resistance genes in clinical and environmental samples due to their high sensitivity, low cost, and compatibility with portable devices.

8.2.1.2 Optical and Fluorescent Biosensors

Optical biosensors are analytical tools that use optical phenomena to identify and measure chemicals and biological materials. One of the most common forms of biosensors is optical, especially those that use Surface Plasmon Resonance (SPR). By monitoring variations in refractive index close to a sensor surface, they enable real-time, label-free identification of analytes like viruses, poisons, and biomarkers. These sensors generate signals proportional to the concentration of the target analyte by utilizing a variety of biorecognition components, such as enzymes, antibodies, and nucleic acids. [15]. High specificity, sensitivity, and the capacity to perform tests without requiring substantial sample preparation are among the benefits of optical biosensors, which makes them appropriate for use in environmental and medical applications [16].

8.2.1.3 Mass-Sensitive Biosensors

Mass-sensitive biosensors, such as quartz crystal microbalances, measure changes in mass on a sensor surface. These are ideal for detecting microbial growth and antibiotic residues in environmental and agricultural samples, providing insights into resistance dynamics in ecosystems [17].

8.2.1.4 Multi-Target and Reconfigurable Biosensors

Recent developments have led to biosensors capable of detecting multiple targets simultaneously. These reconfigurable devices are ideal for complex environments like wastewater or mixed microbial cultures. Their versatility ensures broad applicability across healthcare, agriculture, and environmental surveillance. The Table 8.1 summarizes biosensors used in AMR surveillance.

Table 8.1 Potential biosensors for antimicrobial resistance (AMR) monitoring

Example of biosensor	Type	Working	Reference
E-Si-CRISPR biosensor	Electrochemical biosensor	It employs CRISPR technology to detect methicillin-resistant Staphylococcus aureus (MRSA) without nucleic acid amplification, demonstrating high selectivity even in complex samples like human serum.	[12]
Pathogen detection biosensor	Electrochemical biosensor	Utilizes electrochemical measurement of 16S rRNA to rapidly determine pathogen-antibiotic susceptibility directly from clinical samples, achieving results in approximately 3.5 hours.	[18]
Electrochemical aptasensor for ARGs	Electrochemical biosensor	Uses aptamers that bind specifically to antibiotic resistance genes, generating an electrochemical signal proportional to the concentration of the target, allowing for rapid detection of AMR	[12]
Biochip system for multidrug-resistant TB	Optical biosensor	A rapid biochip system evaluates sputum samples for multidrug-resistant tuberculosis by detecting specific bacterial cultures using optical signals, enhancing diagnostic speed and accuracy.	[18]
Quartz Crystal Microbalance (QCM) sensor	Mass-sensitive biosensor	Measures frequency changes in response to bacterial attachment, allowing real-time monitoring of bacterial growth and antibiotic susceptibility through mass changes, suitable for AMR surveillance.	[13]
TMA biosensor	Electrochemical biosensor	Detects trimethylamine (TMA) in fish freshness by immobilizing flavin-containing monooxygenase on a dissolved oxygen electrode, calibrated against TMA solutions for accurate freshness evaluation.	[19]

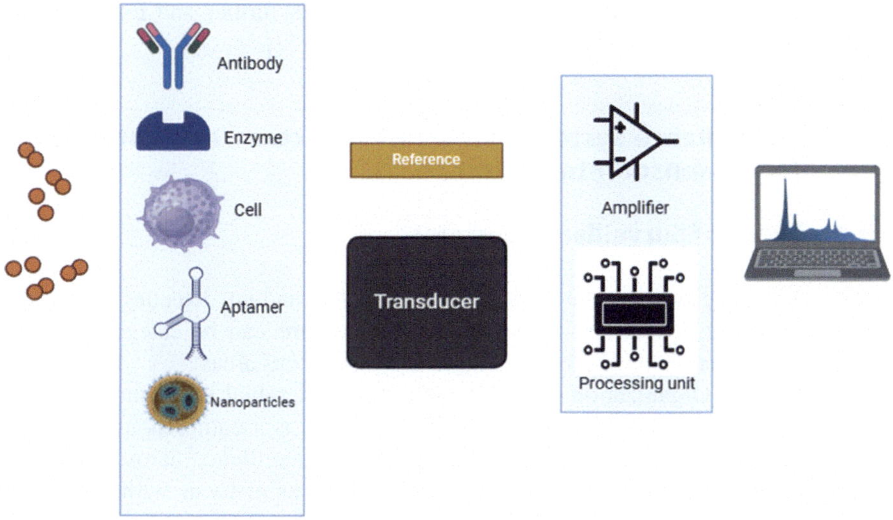

Fig. 8.2 Biosensor consisting of a bioreceptor, transducer, electronic system (amplifier and processor), and display [20]

8.2.2 Key Components of Biosensors

Biosensors typically consist of the following components (Fig. 8.2):

- **Analyte**: A substance of interest whose constituents are being identified or detected.
- **Biorecognition Elements**: Molecules such as enzymes, antibodies, or aptamers that specifically interact with the target analyte.
- **Transducers**: Devices that convert biological interactions into measurable signals, such as electrical or optical outputs.
- **Signal Processing Units**: Tools that amplify and interpret the signal, often incorporating AI for advanced data analysis.

8.2.3 Recent Advances in Biosensor Design and Sensitivity for AMR

Recent advances in biosensors have significantly enhanced the ability to detect AMR rapidly and accurately. Innovations such as electrochemical sensors utilizing DNA probes have emerged as effective tools for identifying antibiotic-resistant pathogens. These sensors offer advantages over traditional methods, including faster response times and lower costs, making them suitable for point-of-care testing. By integrating novel materials, enhancing multiplex detection capabilities, and utilizing advanced molecular techniques, these biosensors provide rapid, accurate, and cost-effective solutions for AMR surveillance. Continued research and development are essential to refine these technologies further and expand their applications in clinical and environmental settings [21, 22].

8.3 Surveillance Systems: Structure, Function, and Potential for Biosensor Integration

8.3.1 Types of Surveillance Systems

AMR surveillance systems play a crucial role in understanding, detecting, and combating the spread of resistant pathogens. These systems can be categorized into several types based on their scope, methodology, and focus areas.

World Health Organization's (WHO) Global Antimicrobial Resistance and Use Surveillance System (GLASS) was launched in 2015, is a comprehensive global surveillance system that aims to standardize AMR surveillance across countries [23]. It encompasses several modules for different areas of focus with respect to AMR surveillance. As of 2022, 127 countries, territories, and areas participate in GLASS, making it a significant global surveillance network [24].

Various countries have established their own national surveillance systems. The United States of America have National Antimicrobial Resistance Monitoring System (NARMS) [25], Norway has Norwegian Surveillance System for Antimicrobial Drug Resistance (NORM) and France has Réseau d'épidémiosurveillance de l'antibiorésistance (RESAPATH).

Surveillance systems can also be classified into specific sectors being monitored. Human Health Surveillance is focused on the monitoring AMR in human pathogens taken form the clinical laboratories and hospitals [26]. This data helps in resistance developed against antibiotics across populations. Animal and Agriculture Surveillances are focused on livestock, poultry and agricultural produce [27]. These help in monitoring changes related to animal feed, veterinary medicine and pesticides to better understand the spread and resistance developed by pathogens through food. Lastly Environmental surveillance systems incorporate monitoring and tracking AMR in soil, water and sewage, to better understand the spread of AMR due to industrial transmission pathways [28, 29].

Passive surveillance systems rely on routine reporting from organizations such as healthcare facilities or animal laboratories, utilizing existing infrastructure to collect data. While they are cost-effective and suitable for monitoring long-term trends, they may suffer from incomplete or delayed data due to reliance on self-reporting. In contrast, active surveillance systems involve proactive efforts, such as deploying public health staff to systematically collect data on target pathogens. These systems offer more comprehensive and timely information but require greater resources, including time, personnel, and funding.

Recognizing the interconnected nature of AMR across human, animal, and environmental sectors, some surveillance systems adopt a One Health approach. These integrated systems aim to provide a more comprehensive understanding of AMR dynamics across different domains [24].

8.3.2 Data Collection and Transmission in Surveillance Networks

Data collection and transmission are crucial components of surveillance networks, encompassing various methods and technologies to gather, process, and disseminate information effectively. These systems play a vital role in monitoring public health, security, and other critical areas.AMR surveillance involves collecting data from diverse sources, including clinical laboratories (microbiology results, antimicrobial susceptibility testing, and pathogen identification), hospitals and clinics (patient records, infection data, and prescribed antimicrobial treatments), community surveillance (outpatient settings and public health campaigns), animal and food sources (livestock, aquaculture, and food products), and environmental monitoring (water, soil, and waste). Passive surveillance relies on self-reported data from physicians, laboratories, death records, disease registries, and hospital records, offering cost-effective monitoring but often lacking completeness and timeliness. In contrast, active surveillance proactively gathers data from targeted sources, such as sentinel sites, serial health surveys, and linked databases, ensuring comprehensive and timely insights but requiring greater resources. Together, these systems provide critical data for understanding and combating antimicrobial resistance.

The transmission of AMR data to surveillance systems involves several sophisticated methods and technologies. Electronic Data Transmission allows clinical laboratories, hospitals, and other data sources to upload microbiology results, antimicrobial susceptibility testing (AST), and infection data directly to centralized surveillance systems using digital platforms, streamlining data collection and minimizing manual entry errors [30, 31]. Automated Reporting Systems, such as Laboratory Information Management Systems (LIMS) and hospital Electronic Health Records (EHRs), automatically generate and share reports in standardized formats, reducing errors and ensuring consistent data across various sources [32]. Centralized Databases like the WHO's Global Antimicrobial Resistance Surveillance System (GLASS) aggregate data from multiple sources to provide a comprehensive analysis of AMR trends globally. Real-Time Reporting mechanisms, such as the California Reportable Disease Information Exchange (CalREDIE), enable rapid responses to emerging AMR patterns by allowing real-time laboratory reporting. Interoperable Networks integrate data from hospitals, community health centers, and environmental monitoring programs into unified systems, offering a more comprehensive view of AMR patterns across different healthcare and environmental settings. Finally, Secure Transmission Channels, using encryption protocols, secure file transfer systems like SFTP [33], and strong authentication measures, ensure data integrity and protect patient confidentiality during transmission.

8.3.3 The Importance of Real-Time Monitoring and Predictive Analytics in AMR Surveillance

AMR has become one of the top public health threats globally, and its rapid spread requires an efficient, data-driven approach to manage and mitigate its effects.

Traditional surveillance methods often fall short in addressing the complexities of AMR, making real-time monitoring and predictive analytics critical for proactive management. These systems often rely on passive data collection, resulting in delays in detecting resistance patterns. Real-time monitoring offers a timel and more accurate picture, while predictive analytics helps forecast potential resistance trends. This proactive approach allows for faster interventions and ensures that resources are allocated more effectively, ultimately improving antimicrobial stewardship while reducing unchecked spreads. Rapid Detection and Response is a key benefit; real-time monitoring allows for quick identification of antimicrobial-resistant infections and the swift implementation of containment strategies. For example, genomics surveillance in hospitals has shown significant success in identifying multidrug-resistant infections and preventing their spread [34].

Improved Decision-Making is another major advantage, as real-time data and predictive insights enable healthcare professionals to make more informed decisions. Tools like WHONET allow for immediate analysis of resistance profiles, ensuring that the most effective treatment strategies are used [2]. Predictive analytics can forecast resistance trends and help healthcare systems allocate resources efficiently. This is particularly useful in Antimicrobial Stewardship, where predictive models can guide optimal drug use, reduce unnecessary antibiotic prescriptions, and help prevent the overuse of antimicrobials, thereby minimizing the development of resistance. Additionally, predictive analytics can guide personalised medicine for the selection of the most effective drug combinations and predicts which patients are at risk of developing resistant infections, contributing to overall AMR burden reduction. Early detection of resistance patterns allows healthcare systems to quickly respond to emerging resistant strains, leading to more effective containment [35]. Reduced AMR burden is achievable through better antimicrobial stewardship practices and more efficient use of resources, which can curb the spread of resistance. These approaches support evidence-based decision-making, improve patient outcomes, and contribute to global health security, making them crucial in the fight against AMR.

8.4 Integrating Biosensors into Surveillance Infrastructures

8.4.1 Frameworks and Architectures for Integration

8.4.1.1 Wired, Wireless, and Hybrid Systems

Biosensor communication systems can be categorized into wired, wireless, and hybrid systems, each offering distinct advantages and challenges. Wired systems involve direct connections between sensors and external devices, ensuring reliable and high-speed data transfer. These systems are ideal for applications requiring low latency and high accuracy but are limited by physical constraints and lack mobility. In contrast, wireless systems utilize technologies such as Bluetooth, Wi-Fi, Zigbee, or LoRa for remote communication, offering greater flexibility and the ability to monitor biosensors in real-time over longer distances [36]. However, they are constrained by bandwidth limitations, potential interference, and security concerns when dealing with HER [37]. Hybrid systems combine both wired and wireless components, providing stability and high-speed processing through wired connections while maintaining flexibility and mobility via wireless transmission. They allow for expansion and easy integration of current infrastructures with wireless nodes making it adaptable and scalable solution. For examples, combining different wireless technologies, such as hardware control with Bluetooth Low Energy (BLE), for efficient data transmission [38].

8.4.1.2 Microfluidic and Wearable Biosensor Technologies

Microfluidic and wearable biosensor technologies have emerged as powerful tools for integrating antimicrobial resistance (AMR) biosensors into surveillance systems. These technologies offer significant advantages in terms of rapid detection, real-time monitoring, and point-of-care diagnostics for AMR.

Microfluidic devices offering several advantages for rapid and efficient detection. The miniaturization aspect of microfluidics, such as lab-on-a-chip devices, allows for point-of-care diagnostics, requiring smaller sample volumes and making the testing process more accessible and efficient [39]. These devices enable fast antibiotic susceptibility testing (AST), significantly reducing testing time from the typical 16–20 h to just 4–5 h [40]. Furthermore, microfluidic platforms facilitate multiplexed detection, enabling the simultaneous analysis of multiple biomarkers, which enhances comprehensive AMR surveillance. These systems are also capable of precise control over the testing process, such as generating accurate antibiotic dilutions comparable to current clinical standards [39, 41].

Wearable biosensors offer continuous, non-invasive monitoring of biomarkers, making them an ideal tool for long-term surveillance [42]. The non-invasive nature of wearable biosensors allows analysis of various biofluids, such as sweat, tears, and saliva, which are less intrusive than blood samples and more suitable for frequent monitoring [43]. Wearable biosensors are also being integrated with smart technologies, including Artificial Intelligiance (AI), machine learning, and IoT, which can further enhance the surveillance capabilities of AMR monitoring systems. This integration also promotes real-time data analysis and predictive analytics, providing healthcare providers with timely insights [39]. The integration of microfluidic and wearable biosensors for AMR surveillance focuses on improving efficiency, accessibility, and scalability. Smartphone integration allows biosensors to use smartphones' processing power for immediate results and data sharing [39, 44], while cloud-based systems enable real-time AMR monitoring across clinical settings. Incorporating AMR biosensors into the IoT facilitates comprehensive monitoring and data analysis. Integrating these technologies enables rapid, continuous, and non-invasive AMR surveillance, enhancing antimicrobial stewardship and treatment.

8.4.2 Communication Protocols (e.g., Bluetooth, Wi-Fi, IoT, and 5G)

The integration of biosensors into surveillance infrastructures requires selecting the right communication protocols to ensure efficient data transmission and connectivity. The choice of protocol depends on factors like range, power consumption, data rate, and security requirements.

8.4.2.1 Short-Range Protocols

Bluetooth, particularly Bluetooth Low Energy (BLE), is widely used for short-range communication in biosensor applications. BLE typically offers a range of about 50–150 m and a data rate of up to 1 Mbps while maintaining low power consumption, making it ideal for battery-powered devices such as wearable biosensors and point-of-care diagnostics. BLE is especially useful for transmitting small amounts of data from biosensors to smartphones or other gateway devices. Wearable electrochemical sensors often utilize BLE to transfer data to mobile phones for collection and analysis [31]. Wi-Fi is another commonly used protocol for higher bandwidth applications. It has a range of up to 100 m indoors, with data rates reaching several Gbps, depending on the standard [45]. While Wi-Fi generally consumes more power than BLE, it is well-suited for applications that require high-resolution imaging or continuous monitoring, and it allows for easy integration with existing network infrastructures in healthcare settings. Such systems have been utilized for machine learning-enabled, colorimetric microfluidic biosensors for real-time, cloud-based AMR monitoring [63].

8.4.2.2 Long-Range Protocols

For applications that require wider coverage, LoRaWAN (Long Range Wide Area Network) is an ideal choice. With a range of up to 10 km in rural areas and 2–3 km in urban environments, LoRaWAN operates at very low power, making it suitable for battery-operated devices [46]. Its low data rate, ranging from 0.3 to 50 kbps, is sufficient for environmental monitoring or large-scale biosensor networks. Such systems have been tested for network-wide surveillance using electrochemical biosensors for real-time monitoring of inland water quality [64].NB-IoT and LTE-M are cellular IoT technologies that provide wide-area coverage, similar to cellular networks. LTE-M offers data rates of up to 1 Mbps, while NB-IoT supports up to 250 kbps [47]. These protocols are suitable for applications like mobile health monitoring and remote patient surveillance, leveraging existing cellular infrastructure for large-scale biosensor deployment.

8.4.2.3 Specialized Protocols

ZigBee, a protocol often used in mesh networks, is another key player in healthcare applications. It supports a range of 10–100 m and offers a data rate of 250 kbps with low power consumption [46]. Its mesh networking capability makes it ideal for hospital room monitoring. In contrast, 5G is an emerging network technology offering high-speed, low-latency communication. With data rates up to 20 Gbps and latency as low as 1 ms [48], 5G is perfect for real-time remote monitoring. It enables advanced applications real-time analysis of complex biosensor data.

8.4.2.4 Protocol Selection Considerations

When selecting communication protocols for biosensor integration, various factors must be considered. For battery-operated devices, low-power protocols like BLE or LoRaWAN are ideal. High-bandwidth applications, require Wi-Fi or 5G. Long-range protocols, such as LoRaWAN or cellular IoT, are essential for large-area deployment. Security is also a crucial consideration, with protocols featuring robust encryption and authentication mechanisms necessary for protecting sensitive health data. Additionally, interoperability with existing systems and devices is important to ensure seamless integration and operation.

8.4.3 Data Fusion Techniques: Combining Biosensor Data with Other Surveillance Data Sources

Biosensors generate valuable health data by integrating with advanced technologies. Cloud-based analytics enable remote storage and real-time analysis for early disease detection. IoT connectivity ensures seamless communication for continuous monitoring, while Healthcare IoT (H-IoT) uses wearable sensors for personalized care. AI and Machine Learning (ML) a analyse patterns for accurate diagnostics, and time series analysis tracks health trends for chronic disease management. Blockchain secures data and enables efficient sharing [49]. These technologies provide continuous, actionable insights. Advanced data fusion techniques, such as feature-level fusion (combining sensor features) and decision-level fusion (integrating sensor outputs), enhance health monitoring and prediction, including AMR-related diseases.

Biosensor data will significantly enhance established AMR surveillance networks, such as WHO's GLASS, the US NARMS, and the European EARS-Net. By providing rapid, real-time data on antimicrobial resistance, biosensors will complement traditional surveillance methods, ensuring faster detection and a more comprehensive understanding of resistance trends. These systems will leverage biosensor data to augment their existing data sources, enhancing global monitoring efforts. Biosensor data will complement conventional culture-based methods by offering quicker initial results, reducing the time required to identify resistant pathogens. Biosensors will also enhance detection sensitivity, particularly when bacterial loads are low, ensuring that even subtle cases of resistance are identified [50]. Additionally, continuous biosensor monitoring in clinical settings will provide ongoing insights, which will be valuable for managing patient care and guiding treatment decisions.

Biosensor data will be combined with clinical information for more detailed analysis of AMR trends. By correlating resistance patterns with patient outcomes, it will be possible to identify risk factors associated with AMR infections. This integration will help inform clinical decision-making and strengthen antibiotic stewardship programs, leading to more targeted and effective interventions. Advanced data analysis techniques such as machine learning (ML) and artificial intelligence (AI) will play a pivotal role in interpreting complex biosensor data. These techniques will develop predictive models for the emergence and spread of AMR, identify novel patterns in resistance, and enhance early warning systems for detecting new threats [51]. The application of AI and ML to biosensor data will support faster and more accurate forecasting of AMR trends.

Additionally, a few challenges will need to be addressed for effective fusion. For biosensor data to be effectively integrated into AMR surveillance systems, standardization will be the key. Developing common protocols for data interpretation and sharing will help create a unified framework. Quality control measures will also need to be established to ensure the reliability of biosensor-generated data. Compliance with data protection regulations, such as GDPR and HIPAA, will need to be prioritized to safeguard patient confidentiality [52]. Additionally, enabling secure data sharing across surveillance networks will allow for collaboration without compromising data integrity or privacy. Biosensor results will need to be compared with traditional gold-standard methods to ensure accuracy and reliability. Moreover, developing guidelines for integrating biosensor data into clinical and public health decision-making processes will ensure that this data is used effectively to inform actions and policies for controlling AMR.

8.5 Applications of Biosensors in AMR Surveillance

8.5.1 Public Health Surveillance

8.5.1.1 Pandemic Preparedness and Response

The pandemic highlighted one of the success stories of rapid diagnostics technologies which realigned and improved public health responses. Rapid antigen testing kits' effectiveness in early detection and intervention has been illuminating and achievable in decentralized resource-restricted situations, particularly in India [53]. Similarly, these technologies can be easily inclined toward the surveillance of AMR, which is currently posing a threat to global health. Rapid results within minutes together with their scalability facilitates decentralized and mass testing fundamental for detection and containment of outbreak as well as optimisation of treatment [53]. The Indian AMRSN and WHO GLASS highlight the need for systematic collection of data and continuous monitoring in real-time. Integration of biosensors with these platforms enables the quick detection of pathogens and provides efficient data handling that enhances early reporting of patterns. These technologies can disrupt chains of transmission, decrease healthcare costs, and strefit with stratified diagnostic models used during COVID-19 [30, 54].

8.5.1.2 Antibiotic Stewardship in Clinical Settings

Microbial resistance to multiple antibiotics resulting from the misuse and overuse of antibiotics in the healthcare and agricultural sectors is a threat to global health, such examples are MDR, including MRSA and CRE [55, 56]. Strategies for stewardship must promote the appropriate use of antibiotics to decrease AMR rates, improve patients' quality of life, and decrease Infections. Technologies like biosensors can bring such changes in stewardship practices. It allows the fast identification of microorganisms, ARGs, and antibiotic levels in clinical specimens removing the need and drawback of culture-based methods [12]. Another example of biosensors are electrochemical platforms that successfully identify pathogens and antimicrobial susceptibility testing (AST) within hours; hence, supporting appropriate clinical judgments and limiting the use of broad-spectrum antibiotics [18]. Applying antibiotic stewardship in parallel with efficient diagnostic tools works on the principle of One-Health, linking human, animal, and environmental health to treat AMR. Clinical care environments must support and provide the guidelines and technologies that will help to remove AMR and save antibiotics for future generations [12, 57].

8.5.2 Environmental Monitoring for AMR

8.5.2.1 Wastewater Surveillance as an Early Warning System

Wastewater surveillance can be defined as the process of identifying pathogens, AMR, and public health biomarkers in wastewater. For example, recently, the identification of SARS-CoV-2 in sewage has predicted the emergence of clinical COVID-19 cases. In a comparable fashion, biosensors detecting AMR genes such as mecA in hospital sewages lit up the dissemination of resistant bacteria. These insights show how WBE successfully and inexpensively provides real-time data that can identify an emerging health threat and inform the public health response, making WBE a powerful approach to monitoring population health and controlling the spread of diseases [58, 59].

8.5.2.2 Agriculture and Livestock Surveillance for AMR Spread

CIPARS (Canada) and DANMAP (Denmark) are the known official organizations that link AMU and AMR in production animals to human health [60]. CIPARS in farm animal's surveys AMU and AMR in retail meat, but DANMAP covers for pathogens such as the E. Coil and has endorsed policies such as the Denmark no-use policy on antibiotic growth promoters [60]. AMR is very significant in agriculture and livestock since farmers use antibiotics in feed for disease control treatment and promotion of growth hence depleting human health and food security. Biosensors provide quick and affordable ways to identify antibiotics and resistant bacteria in milk and soil, allowing for on-site AMR monitoring [61, 62].

8.6 Data Analysis and Interpretation in Biosensor-Driven AMR Surveillance

The integration of biosensors into AMR surveillance generates vast amounts of data, necessitating advanced analytical tools for meaningful interpretation. Big data platforms, artificial intelligence (AI), machine learning (ML), and blockchain technology play pivotal roles in this context.

8.6.1 Big Data Platforms for Centralized Analysis, Visualization and Actionable Insights of Biosensor Data

Integrating biosensor outputs with big data platforms has transformed antimicrobial resistance (AMR) surveillance by enhancing efficiency, credibility, and actionable insights. These platforms adhere to the One Health principle, consolidating data from human, animal, and environmental sources into unified systems for comprehensive monitoring and prediction [60]. In India, the i-AMRSS (Indian Council of Medical Research Antimicrobial Resistance Surveillance System) centralizes hospital data, employing open-source technologies to standardize testing and enable evidence-based policy interventions [63]. At the global level, WHO's GLASS (Global Antimicrobial Resistance and Use Surveillance System) harmonizes AMR data across countries, supporting cross-country comparisons and international collaboration [57, 60].

Advanced biosensors, such as CRISPR-based and fluorescence-based technologies, provide real-time outputs that feed into these platforms, allowing identification of resistance trends, prediction of hotspots, and informed decision-making [64]. Platforms like PATHFINDER integrate diverse datasets from hospitals, agriculture, and wastewater, using machine learning algorithms to normalize testing, generate MIC plots, and visualize resistance in pathogens like *E. coli* [65]. Flowchart of Big Data Platforms for Centralized Analysis, visualization and actionable insights of Biosensor Data is shown in Fig. 8.3.

Visualization tools, including geospatial maps, dashboards, and heat maps, facilitate real-time monitoring. Programs like CIPARS and DANMAP could utilize biosensor data to link antibiotic use with resistance markers, ensuring rapid detection of ARGs and contaminants. These platforms empower evidence-based interventions, strengthen decision-making, and are pivotal in combating AMR globally [60, 66].

8.6.2 Predictive and Prescriptive Analytics with AI and Machine Learning

AI and ML are used in AMR surveillance to predict resistance trends and guide actions to control and manage antimicrobial resistance effectively. Using machine

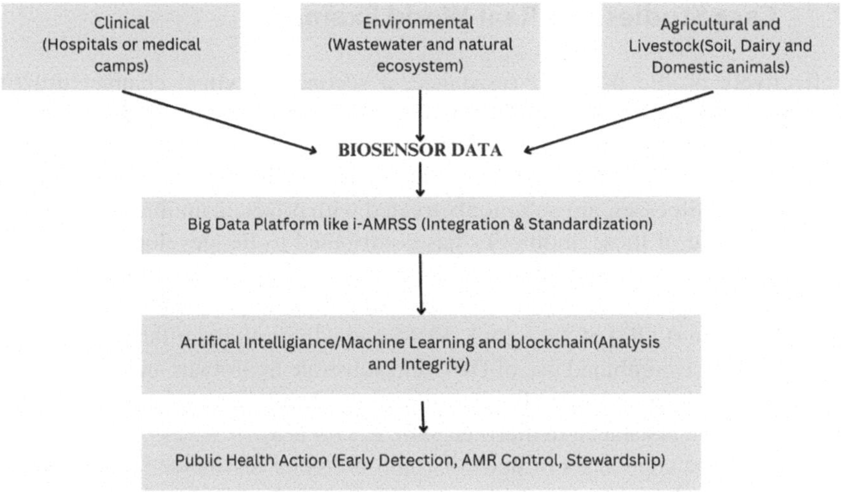

Fig. 8.3 Big data platforms for Biosensor data

learning models like PATHFINDER which is capable of running through genomic information to predict resistance in bacteria for example *E. coli* and *P. aeruginosa* [65]. These biomarkers are discovered through deep learning and prescriptive analysis where gene database and artificial intelligence are incorporated for producing the treatment for antimicrobial stewardship [67, 68]. In biosensor data analysis, pattern recognition algorithms detect ARGs, and thus applying mitigation measures in agriculture. AI also identifies areas of resistance on multi-omics and geographical densities to facilitate faster implementation of decisions backed by data against AMR [67, 69].

8.6.3 Blockchain for Data Integrity, Privacy, and Traceability

Blockchain has the possibility to revolutionise AMR surveillance through security, privacy, and auditability. Its decentralized system offers an unalterable record of data on AMR and maintains the trust of different stakeholders. With pertinent health records information protected by encryption, the respective patient information remains protected while only authorize researchers and health authorities can access it. Furthermore, tracking of information within the healthcare chain increases openness of drug utilization and resistance, as well as allowing for appropriate and prompt corrective actions. Combination of the blockchain with AI and IoT also enhances AMR surveillance, using real-time data transfer and analysis for practical and efficient healthcare management [70–72].

8.7 Case Studies and Real-World Examples

To effectively profile β-lactam resistance, a second analytical channel utilizing differential-pulse voltammetry (DPV) was employed. This method enabled the measurement of the hydrolyzed product of nitrocefin, providing precise characterization of enzymatic activity. Diarrheagenic *E. coli* infections, a frequent cause of gastrointestinal illnesses, are commonly treated with β-lactam antibiotics. However, the extensive use of these antibiotics has contributed to the development of resistance, largely due to the production of β-lactamase enzymes. In a study, the detection of β-lactamase activity was achieved with a high degree of sensitivity, with a limit of detection (LOD) of 3.6 ng/mL ±1.65 and a limit of quantification (LOQ) of 10 ng/mL ±4. The combined use of DPV and substrate hydrolysis analysis provides a robust approach to understanding resistance mechanisms and supports efforts to combat antibiotic resistance in diarrheagenic *E. coli* [73].

To address the challenges of detecting antimicrobial resistance (AMR) in complex matrices, such as dairy products, a study employed a novel approach involving molecularly imprinted nanostructures (nanoMIPs). These nanostructures were meticulously engineered to serve as high-affinity synthetic receptors. When coupled with a surface plasmon resonance (SPR) sensor, this innovative design facilitated the precise analysis of glycopeptide antibiotics, specifically vancomycin, in milk samples. The nanoMIP-SPR biosensor demonstrated remarkable sensitivity and accuracy in quantifying vancomycin levels. Two distinct assay methodologies were employed: a direct assay, which achieved a limit of detection (LOD) of 4.1 ng/mL, and a competitive assay, which yielded an LOD of 17.7 ng/mL. These values underscore the sensor's capability to detect even trace amounts of antibiotics, a critical requirement for effective AMR surveillance. Furthermore, the recovery rates for both methods ranged between 85% and 110%, with relative standard deviations (RSDs) consistently below 7%, highlighting the method's reliability and reproducibility. A key advantage of this system lies in the exceptional binding affinity between the Nanomed receptors and the target molecule, vancomycin. The dissociation constant (1.8×10^{-9} M) indicates a binding strength that surpasses not only traditional synthetic receptors but also many naturally occurring receptors. This superior performance ensures more precise and consistent detection, making it a highly effective tool for AMR monitoring [74].

8.8 Challenges and Future Scope

Biosensors used for antimicrobial resistance diagnostics need further development before clinical use because their reliability and effectiveness should undergo detailed validation. The complete evaluation of biosensors through clinical trials under various patient populations becomes essential for determining their performance when using different sample types across multiple clinical settings. The tests evaluate nano-enabled biosensor abilities regarding AMR detection and antibiotic treatment decision support [75].

Biosensors continue to be studied because they demonstrate their capability to create individualized antimicrobial treatments which results in superior clinical results. The scientific research on biosensors demonstrates their potential to help clinicians deliver specific antimicrobial treatments which lead to better healthcare results. A number of challenges must be resolved in order for biosensors to implement effectively in standard clinical practice. These include:

1. **Standardization of methodologies**—Standardization of methodologies demands the creation of uniform testing protocols that also enables criteria validation to achieve platform performance consistency. Research collaborations and regulatory standards need to unite criteria for assessing biosensor-based AMR diagnostic systems.
2. **Scalability and large-scale production**—Commercial manufacturing needs efficient scalable fabrication processes to transition laboratory biosensors from development to production while maintaining high sensitivity along with specificity. Microfabrication and nanotechnology development enables better techniques for bulk biosensor manufacturing methods.
3. **Cost-effectiveness and affordability**—High production expenses related to biosensor development create barriers against their mass adoption because of unaffordable prices. By using affordable materials along with automated production methods and streamlined manufacturing practices these diagnostic solutions will become more affordable for settings with limited resources.
4. **Regulatory compliance and approval**—The safety reliability and efficiency of biosensors needs to satisfy regulatory framework requirements for approval. Regulatory agencies become supportive when developers interact early in device production and follow confirmed diagnostic device standards for market approval.
5. **Clinical validation and real-world applicability**—The application of AMR biosensors depends on running extensive clinical tests that prove their accuracy for detecting infections in different testing environments. Laboratory research across multiple medical sites with patients from different backgrounds will create reliable data for biosensor diagnostic effectiveness [76].

The current challenges need to be resolved for biosensors to gain wide acceptance in healthcare environments. Clinical implementation of biosensors requires combined work from researchers with clinicians and regulatory bodies to solve current issues while proving clinical worth. Biosensors will change the future of AMR diagnostics when their operational challenges are solved because they will generate precise results and actionable information. [77].

8.9 Conclusion

The combination of biosensors within surveillance infrastructure delivers a revolutionary method for managing antimicrobial resistance (AMR). Standard diagnostic procedures take more than 24 h for complete results, but biosensors manage diagnostics in a period ranging from minutes to hours. Fast response times remain essential for medical staff to make appropriate tacit decisions regarding drug therapy while treating bacterial infections from resistant microorganisms. The monitoring of AMR becomes substantially enhanced through biosensors because they deliver rapid and sensitive and cost-efficient detection capabilities in clinical and environmental areas. The developed improvement presents possibilities to enhance both patient care results and public health intervention effectiveness. Biosensors act as an innovative integration technology to surveil antibiotic resistance through solving time-consuming and expense-intensive traditional diagnostic approaches. Biosensors enable fast and budget-friendly detection of antibiotics together with their resistance genes and microbial activities which allows healthcare decisions to be made quickly while enhancing health security policies.

References

1. Chin KW, Michelle Tiong HL, Luang-In V, Ma NL (2023) An overview of antibiotic and antibiotic resistance. Environ Adv 11:100331
2. Miethke M, Pieroni M, Weber T, Brönstrup M, Hammann P, Halby L et al (2021) Towards the sustainable discovery and development of new antibiotics. Nat Rev Chem 5(10):726–749
3. Sable H, Kumar V, Singh V, Rustagi S, Chaudhary V, Pandit S (2024) Review—Nanosystems-enhanced electrochemical biosensors for precision in one health management. J Electrochem Soc [Internet] [cited 2024 Mar 28]; Available from: http://iopscience.iop.org/article/10.1149/1945-7111/ad32a1
4. Guliy OI, Evstigneeva SS, Karavaeva OA (2023) Antimicrobial resistance and current methods for its detection. Front Biosci-Elite 15(3):19
5. Chaudhary V (2025) Perspective—rising era of green semiconductors at nanoscale: challenges and prospects. J Electrochem Soc 172(1):017501–017501
6. Chaudhary V (2022) Prospects of green nanotechnology for efficient management of neurodegenerative diseases. Front Nanotechnol 4:1055708–1055708
7. Laxminarayan R, Duse A, Wattal C, Zaidi AKM, Wertheim HFL, Sumpradit N et al (2013) Antibiotic resistance-the need for global solutions. Lancet Infect Dis 13(12):1057–1098
8. Singh V, Kasana E, Batra J, Sable H, Saxena R (2022) Antimicrobial resistance: mechanisms, screening techniques and biosensors
9. Boodhoo N, Shoja Doost J, Sharif S (2024) Biosensors for monitoring, detecting, and tracking dissemination of poultry-borne bacterial pathogens along the poultry value chain: a review. Anim Open Access J MDPI 14(21):3138
10. Chaudhary V, Lucky L, Sable H, Bhalla N (2025) Interdisciplinary approach to monkeypox prevention: integrating nanobiosensors, nanovaccines, artificial intelligence, visual arts, and social sciences. Small Struct 6(7):2400647–2400647
11. Chauhan N, Sankhla MS, Sharma A, Sable H, Sharma T (2025) Nanotechnology-enhanced detection of illicit drugs: development of Nano sensors for rapid identification in liquid media. J Electrochem Soc 172(7):077505–077505
12. Magnano San Lio R, Barchitta M, Maugeri A, La Rosa MC, Favara G, Agodi A (2023) Updates on developing and applying biosensors for the detection of microorganisms, antimicrobial resistance genes and antibiotics: a scoping review. Front Public Health [Internet] [cited 2024 Dec 19];11. Available from: https://www.frontiersin.org/journals/public-health/articles/10.3389/fpubh.2023.1240584/full
13. Reynoso EC, Laschi S, Palchetti I, Torres E (2021) Advances in antimicrobial resistance monitoring using sensors and biosensors: a review. Chemosensors 9(8):232
14. Cho IH, Kim DH, Park S (2020) Electrochemical biosensors: perspective on functional nanomaterials for on-site analysis. Biomater Res 24(1):6

15. Damborský P, Švitel J, Katrlík J (2016) Optical biosensors. Essays Biochem 60(1):91–100
16. Pashchenko O, Shelby T, Banerjee T, Santra S (2018) A comparison of optical, electrochemical, magnetic, and colorimetric point-of-care biosensors for infectious disease diagnosis. ACS Infect Dis 4(8):1162–1178
17. Hoß SG, Bendas G (2017) Mass-sensitive biosensor systems to determine the membrane interaction of analytes. Methods Mol Biol Clifton NJ 1520:145–157
18. Mach KE, Mohan R, Baron EJ, Shih MC, Gau V, Wong PK et al (2011) A biosensor platform for rapid antimicrobial susceptibility testing directly from clinical samples. J Urol 185(1):148–153
19. Rout P, Chakraborty C (2020) The commercial application of biosensors as an analytical device. Int J Curr Microbiol Appl Sci 9(5):864–880
20. Naresh V, Lee N (2021) A review on biosensors and recent development of nanostructured materials-enabled biosensors. Sensors 21(4):1109
21. Chaudhary V, Awan HTA, Khalid M, Bhadola P, Tandon R, Khosla A (2023) Progress in engineering interlayer space modulated MXenes to architect next-generation airborne pollutant sensors. Sens Actuators B Chem 379:133225–133225
22. Taha BA, Ahmed NM, Talreja RK, Haider AJ, Al Mashhadany Y, Al-Jubouri Q et al (2024 Jun) Synergizing nanomaterials and artificial intelligence in advanced optical biosensors for precision antimicrobial resistance diagnosis. ACS Synth Biol 13(6):1600–1620
23. Global Antimicrobial Resistance and Use Surveillance System (GLASS) [Internet]. [cited 2024 Dec 19]. Available from: https://www.who.int/initiatives/glass
24. Tang KWK, Millar BC, Moore JE (2023) Antimicrobial Resistance (AMR). Br J Biomed Sci 80:11387
25. CDC. National Antimicrobial Resistance Monitoring System for Enteric Bacteria (NARMS) (2024) [cited 2024 Dec 19]. About the National Antimicrobial Resistance Monitoring System (NARMS). Available from: https://www.cdc.gov/narms/about/index.html
26. Lim C, Miliya T, Chansamouth V, Aung MT, Karkey A, Teparrukkul P et al (2020) Automating the generation of antimicrobial resistance surveillance reports: proof-of-concept study involving seven hospitals in seven countries. J Med Internet Res 22(10):e19762
27. Keck N, Treilles M, Gordoncillo M, Ivette OLI, Dauphin G, Dorado-Garcia A et al (2022) A systematic approach toward progressive improvement of national antimicrobial resistance surveillance systems in food and agriculture sectors. Front Vet Sci 9:1057040
28. Hart A, Warren J, Wilkinson H, Schmidt W (2023 Mar) Environmental surveillance of antimicrobial resistance (AMR), perspectives from a national environmental regulator in 2023. Euro Surveill Bull Eur Sur Mal Transm Eur Commun Dis Bull 28(11):2200367
29. Sable H, Tripathy DB (2021) (PDF) A review on comparative analysis on different Sort of physiological and behavioral biometric framework. Int J Adv Res Innov:52–56
30. Robillard DW, Sundermann AJ, Raux BR, Prinzi AM (2024) Navigating the network: a narrative overview of AMR surveillance and data flow in the United States. Antimicrob Steward Healthc Epidemiol ASHE 4(1):e55
31. Ghani S, Khan N, Sable H, Yao F, Shafiq M (2025) Computational techniques for enhancing PK/PD modeling and simulation and ADMET prediction. In: Computational methods in medicinal chemistry, pharmacology, and toxicology, pp 153–174
32. Musa K, Okoliegbe I, Abdalaziz T, Aboushady AT, Stelling J, Gould IM (2023) Laboratory surveillance, quality management, and its role in addressing antimicrobial resistance in Africa: a narrative review. Antibiot Basel Switz 12(8):1313
33. Neves A, Walther D, Martin-Campos T, Barbie V, Bertelli C, Blanc D et al (2023) The Swiss pathogen surveillance platform – towards a nation-wide one health data exchange platform for bacterial, viral and fungal genomics and associated metadata. Microb Genomics 9(5):mgen001001
34. Jauneikaite E, Baker KS, Nunn JG, Midega JT, Hsu LY, Singh SR et al (2023) Genomics for antimicrobial resistance surveillance to support infection prevention and control in health-care facilities. Lancet Microbe 4(12):e1040–e1046

35. Ali T, Ahmed S, Aslam M (2023) Artificial intelligence for antimicrobial resistance prediction: challenges and opportunities towards practical implementation. Antibiot Basel Switz. 12(3):523
36. Famá F, Faria JN, Portugal D (2022) An IoT-based interoperable architecture for wireless biomonitoring of patients with sensor patches. Internet Things 19:100547
37. Bakar K, Zuhra F, Isyaku B, Sulaiman S (2023) A review on the immediate advancement of the internet of things in wireless telecommunications. IEEE Access 11:21020–21048
38. Uddin R, Koo I (2024) Real-time remote patient monitoring: a review of biosensors integrated with multi-hop IoT systems via cloud connectivity. Appl Sci 14(5):1876
39. Apoorva S, Nguyen NT, Sreejith KR (2024) Recent developments and future perspectives of microfluidics and smart technologies in wearable devices. Lab Chip 24(7):1833–1866
40. Nguyen AV, Yaghoobi M, Azizi M, Davaritouchaee M, Simpson KW, Abbaspourrad A (2023) Ladder-shaped microfluidic system for rapid antibiotic susceptibility testing. Commun Eng 2(1):1–12
41. Harsh S, Vaishali K, Vandana S. B2-microglobulin biomarkers' roles in assessing cadmium toxicity
42. Wang Q, Li S, Chen J, Yang L, Qiu Y, Du Q et al (2023) A novel strategy for therapeutic drug monitoring: application of biosensors to quantify antimicrobials in biological matrices. J Antimicrob Chemother 78(11):2612–2629
43. Islam T, Washington P (2024) Non-invasive biosensing for healthcare using artificial intelligence: a semi-systematic review. Biosensors 14(4):183
44. Chaudhary V, Kaushik A, Furukawa H, Khosla A (2022) Review—towards 5th generation AI and IoT driven sustainable intelligent sensors based on 2D MXenes and Borophene. ECS Sens Plus 1(1):013601–013601
45. Doulani K, Adhikari M, Hazra A (2023) Edge-based smart health monitoring device for infectious disease prediction using biosensors. IEEE Sensors J 23:20215–20222
46. Iman U, Zada M, Basir A, Hayat S, Lim YH, Yoo H (2024) IoT-enabled real-time health monitoring via smart textile integration with LoRa technology across diverse environments. IEEE Trans Ind Inform
47. Bhardwaj S, Malik P, Islam T, Gehlot A, Das S, Asha S (2023) A printed monopole antenna for next generation internet of things: narrow-band internet of things (NB-IoT). Prog Electromagn Res C 138:117–129
48. Cabanillas-Carbonell M, Pérez-Martínez J, A. Yáñez J (2023) 5G Technology in the Digital Transformation of healthcare, a systematic review. Sustainability 15(4):3178
49. Kumar M, Kumar A, Verma S, Bhattacharya P, Ghimire D, Kim S-h et al (2023) Healthcare internet of things (H-IoT): current trends, future prospects, applications, challenges, and security issues. Electronics 12(9):2050
50. Jegan R, Anusuya K, v. (2018) Biosensor-based feature extraction and physiological parameters measurement for biomedical applications. Int J Biomed Eng Technol 28(1):67–80
51. Smith AA, Li R, Tse ZTH (2023) Reshaping healthcare with wearable biosensors. Sci Rep 13(1):4998
52. Said A, Yahyaoui A, Abdellatif T (2024) HIPAA and GDPR compliance in IoT healthcare systems. 198–209
53. Kanaujia R, Ghosh A, Mohindra R, Singla V, Goyal K, Gudisa R et al (2021) Rapid antigen detection kit for the diagnosis of SARS-CoV-2 – are we missing asymptomatic patients? Indian J Med Microbiol 39(4):457–461
54. Walia K, Madhumathi J, Veeraraghavan B, Chakrabarti A, Kapil A, Ray P et al (2019) Establishing antimicrobial resistance surveillance & research network in India: journey so far. Indian J Med Res 149(2):164–179
55. Browne AJ, Chipeta MG, Haines-Woodhouse G, Kumaran EPA, Hamadani BHK, Zaraa S et al (2021 Dec) Global antibiotic consumption and usage in humans, 2000-18: a spatial modelling study. Lancet Planet Health 5(12):e893–e904
56. Larsson DGJ, Flach CF (2022) Antibiotic resistance in the environment. Nat Rev Microbiol 20(5):257–269

57. Frost I, Kapoor G, Craig J, Liu D, Laxminarayan R (2021) Status, challenges and gaps in antimicrobial resistance surveillance around the world. J Glob Antimicrob Resist 25:222–226
58. Mao K, Zhang H, Pan Y, Yang Z (2021) Biosensors for wastewater-based epidemiology for monitoring public health. Water Res 191:116787
59. Chen B, He J, Tian K, Qu J, Hong L, Lin Q et al (2024) Research Progress on detection of pathogens in medical wastewater by electrochemical biosensors. Molecules 29(15):3534
60. Delpy L, Astbury CC, Aenishaenslin C, Ruckert A, Penney TL, Wiktorowicz M et al (2024) Integrated surveillance systems for antibiotic resistance in a one health context: a scoping review. BMC Public Health 24(1):1–21
61. Goel P, Vishweswaraiah RH, Kumar N (2022) Spore-based innovative paper-strip biosensor for the rapid detection of ß-lactam group in milk. Sci Rep 12(1):1–13
62. Zhou C, Pan Y, Ge S, Coulon F, Yang Z (2021) Rapid methods for antimicrobial resistance diagnosis in contaminated soils for effective remediation strategy. TrAC Trends Anal Chem 137:116203
63. Kaur J, Dhama AS, Buttolia H, Kaur J, Walia K, Ohri V et al (2021) ICMR'S antimicrobial resistance surveillance system (i-AMRSS): a promising tool for global antimicrobial resistance surveillance. JAC-Antimicrob Resist 3(1):dlab023
64. Rathore P, Basnet A, Kilonzo-Nthenge A, Dumenyo K, Yadegari Z, Taheri A (2024) Rapid detection of pathogenic E. coli based on CRISPR Cas system. Front Microbiol [Internet]. [cited 2024 Dec 19];15. Available from: https://www.frontiersin.org/journals/microbiology/articles/10.3389/fmicb.2024.1423478/full;
65. Agboeze T, Daramola O, Akomolafe A, Adedeji R, Markwei J (2024) Wellcome Open Research | Open Access Publishing Platform. [cited 2024 Dec 19]. A predictive algorithm for the analysis of AMR trends and …. Available from: https://wellcomeopenresearch.org/articles/9-274/v1
66. Jarocki VM, Cummins ML, Donato CM, Howden BP, Djordjevic SP (2024) A one health approach for the genomic surveillance of AMR. Microbiol Aust 45(2):63–67
67. Kolluru VK, Nuthakki Y, Koganti S, Chintakunta AN (2024) Use of predictive analytics in antimicrobial resistance: a review. Cogniz J Multidiscip Stud 4(1):404–414
68. Kapadia V, Wadhwani A, Begum R, Ponnusankar S, Mohadeb P, Gujadhur M (2024) A step towards combating antimicrobial resistance: global prescriptive and programmes—a review. Biosci Biotechnol Res Asia 21(3):877–892
69. Lu N, Chen J, Rao Z, Guo B, Xu Y (2023) Recent advances of biosensors for detection of multiple antibiotics. Biosensors 13(9):850
70. Sun H, Hu W, Wei Y, Hao Y (2024) Drawing on the development experiences of infectious disease surveillance systems around the world. China CDC Wkly 6(41):1065–1074
71. Chattu VK, Nanda A, Chattu SK, Kadri SM, Knight AW (2019) The emerging role of blockchain technology applications in routine disease surveillance systems to strengthen global health security. Big Data Cogn Comput 3(2):25
72. Umrao D, Mathur A, Patel CS, Awasthi A, Tiwari A (2022) Blockchain technology in the health sector. Int J Health Sci 6(S1):12485–12495
73. Gunasekaran D, Rostovsky I, Taussig D, Bar-Am T, Wine Y, Sal-Man N et al (2024) A dual-channel electrochemical biosensor enables concurrent detection of pathogens and antibiotic resistance. Biosens Bioelectron 257:116314
74. Altintas Z (2018) Surface plasmon resonance based sensor for the detection of glycopeptide antibiotics in milk using rationally designed nanoMIPs. Sci Rep 8(1):11222
75. Ho D, Quake SR, McCabe ERB, Chng WJ, Chow EK, Ding X et al (2020) Enabling technologies for personalized and precision medicine. Trends Biotechnol 38(5):497–518
76. Shrivastava S, Trung TQ, Lee NE (2020) Recent progress, challenges, and prospects of fully integrated mobile and wearable point-of-care testing systems for self-testing. Chem Soc Rev 49(6):1812–1866
77. Akhlaghi AA, Kaur H, Adhikari BR, Soleymani L (2024) Editors' choice—challenges and opportunities for developing electrochemical biosensors with commercialization potential in the point-of-care diagnostics market. ECS Sens Plus 3(1):011601

Leveraging Geospatial Analysis to Understand the AMR Crisis in Remote and Mountainous Regions: Lessons from Northern Pakistan

9

Rizwan Shahid, Kashif Ali Khan, Bashir Ullah,
Stefania Bertazzon, and Zul Kamal

9.1 Introduction & Background

AMR poses a critical threat to global public health, causing an estimated 1.27 million deaths in 2019 and 4.95 million in 2020. The misuse and overuse of antimicrobials across human health, agriculture, and veterinary medicine aggravate this crisis, rendering standard treatments increasingly ineffective. The economic impact of AMR is staggering, with projected global costs of up to $3.4 trillion annually by 2030 [1]. Recognizing the urgency, global leaders at the 2024 UN General Assembly set ambitious targets to reduce bacterial AMR deaths by 10% by 2030. Initiatives such as the World Antimicrobial Resistance Awareness Week (WAAW) aim to improve understanding and promote best practices across sectors, while antimicrobial stewardship programs focused on optimizing antibiotic use to curb resistance [2–5].

R. Shahid (✉)
University of Calgary, Calgary, AB, Canada

O'Brien Institute for Public Health, Calgary, AB, Canada

Primary Care Alberta, Calgary, AB, Canada
e-mail: rizwan.shahid1@ucalgary.ca

K. A. Khan · B. Ullah
Chongqing University of Chinese Medicines, Chongqing, People's Republic of China

S. Bertazzon
University of Calgary, Calgary, AB, Canada

O'Brien Institute for Public Health, Calgary, AB, Canada

Z. Kamal
Chongqing University of Chinese Medicines, Chongqing, People's Republic of China

Shaheed Benazir Bhutto University, Sheringal, Khyber Pakhtunkhwa, Pakistan

V. Chaudhary, N. Bhalla (eds.), *Biosensors for Tackling Antimicrobial Resistance (AMR)*, https://doi.org/10.1007/978-981-95-9151-0_9

Remote and mountainous regions face unique challenges in managing AMR due to their geographic isolation, limited healthcare access, and reliance on traditional practices. In these areas, self-medication and unsupervised antibiotic use are prevalent, further compounding resistance risks. Socioeconomic factors, including poverty and inadequate resources, worsen the problem, while livestock practices such as improper antibiotic use in animals, serve as additional drivers of AMR [6, 7]. Environmental factors, such as water contamination and proximity to livestock, further contribute to the spread of resistant pathogens [8].

Geospatial analysis provides valuable insights into the spatial dimensions of AMR, helping identify hotspots and patterns of resistance [9]. Geographic Information Systems (GIS) enable researchers to map AMR prevalence, integrate environmental data, and predict future resistance trends. By linking human, animal, and environmental health, GIS supports targeted interventions and policy-making in AMR research. However, challenges such as data availability, underreporting, and variability in microbial resistance dynamics highlight the need for robust, high-resolution spatial data and multidisciplinary collaboration [10–12].

Addressing AMR in remote regions requires context-specific approaches tailored to local practices and environmental conditions. A combination of geospatial tools, surveillance systems, and community education is essential for mitigating the AMR threat, fostering sustainable public health solutions in vulnerable areas worldwide [4, 8, 13].

9.2 Healthcare Landscape in Pakistan

The Pakistani healthcare system comprises both public and private sectors, with the government spending only 1.2% of GDP on healthcare [14], which is comparatively lower than the rest of the world. This underinvestment leads to inefficiencies, limited accessibility, and poor health outcomes, especially in rural areas. The federal and provincial health ministries govern the system, with provincial administrations managing services locally, while the Federal Ministry of National Health Services coordinates national policies. Urban centers have advanced facilities, but rural areas, which comprise 63% of the population [2], often lack basic services and infrastructure.

The country faces a dual burden of disease: high prevalence of communicable diseases like tuberculosis, hepatitis, and malaria, alongside non-communicable diseases such as diabetes and cardiovascular conditions, which account for 60% of total deaths [8, 15]. WHO highlights Pakistan's low doctor-to-population ratio, contributing to a severe healthcare workforce shortage. Government reforms, including the Sehat Insaf Card and vaccination drives, aim to improve service delivery, but challenges like political instability and limited funding hinder progress [16]. NGOs play a critical role in bridging gaps, offering immediate services, and supporting health education and long-term initiatives in underserved communities.

9.2.1 Standard Medical Practice in Pakistan

In Pakistan, standard medical practices are a blend of traditional and modern approaches within a regulatory framework guided by the Pakistan Medical Commission (PMC), health ministries, and provincial health departments. These frameworks aim to regulate medical education, licensing, and practice. However, limited resources, inconsistent guideline implementation, and socioeconomic disparities hinder healthcare quality, particularly in rural areas. Challenges include insufficient financial resources, outdated equipment, and a shortage of trained personnel, leading to gaps in patient care. Continuous Medical Education (CME) programs aim at updating practitioners' knowledge, but uneven implementation creates knowledge gaps, especially in remote regions [17]. Additionally, informal and unqualified healthcare providers complicate the standardization of care, as they often operate outside established safety guidelines.

Government initiatives, such as the Expanded Program on Immunization (EPI), polio eradication campaigns, and maternal and child health programs, strive to enhance care. The COVID-19 pandemic underscored the need for systemic reforms, prompting the adoption of WHO and CDC guidelines, telemedicine, and strengthened emergency preparedness. Improving healthcare standards requires strengthening regulatory bodies like PMC, enhancing workforce training, integrating informal providers, and fostering public-private partnerships to ensure equitable, high-quality care across all regions.

9.2.2 Role of Quackery

Quackery refers to fraudulent healthcare practices carried out by unqualified individuals, posing a significant threat to public health in Pakistan. It accounts for an estimated 70% of healthcare services nationwide [18]. Quacks exploit gaps in the formal healthcare system, particularly in rural and underserved areas where access to qualified medical practitioners is limited. Cultural norms, financial constraints, and inadequate healthcare access drive the acceptance of quacks, especially in remote regions. Traditional healing practices, deeply ingrained in society, often lead patients to bypass standard medical care. Quacks are also usually more affordable compared to licensed professionals, attracting financially constrained patients, despite the risks. This can discourage patients from seeking proper care, increasing the existing burden on healthcare and future challenges. Quackery has serious public health consequences, including increased morbidity and mortality due to unsafe treatments, and the emergence of AMR from inappropriate antibiotic use. Addressing quackery requires stricter enforcement of regulations, improved healthcare access, and public awareness campaigns.

9.2.3 Prevalence of Antibiotics Misuse and AMR

Antibiotic misuse is a major driver of AMR, resulting from practices like overprescription, inappropriate antibiotic selection, and non-adherence to prescribed regimens. This misuse reduces treatment efficacy and accelerates resistance, posing a severe global health threat. In Pakistan, where infectious diseases are highly prevalent, antibiotic misuse is widespread. Approximately 96.1% of patients use antibiotics empirically, without laboratory-confirmed infections [16, 19]. This misuse burdens healthcare systems financially due to longer hospital stays, additional testing, and costly treatments, while patients with resistant infections face higher rates of treatment failure. Addressing this crisis requires coordinated strategies. Strong antibiotic stewardship programs that promote evidence-based prescribing and monitor usage can reduce resistance. Public awareness campaigns are critical to educating people on the risks of misuse and the importance of following prescribed regimens [6, 12]. Additionally, stricter regulations on antibiotic sales can limit over-the-counter access without prescriptions. Enhanced national surveillance systems can also track usage patterns and guide policy decisions effectively. These measures can collectively mitigate the AMR burden and safeguard public health.

9.3 Geospatial Methods in AMR Research

Geospatial techniques are transforming the landscape of AMR research by enabling spatial visualization, analysis, and prediction of resistance patterns and related factors. It provides robust tools to link AMR with demographic, environmental, and healthcare infrastructure variables, offering insights into the factors driving AMR across different settings. This integration helps to inform evidence-based interventions in both urban and remote regions.

GIS has been pivotal in public health, supporting disease mapping, outbreak monitoring, and resource allocation. In AMR research, it links antibiotic resistance to socioeconomic, environmental, and healthcare factors like population density, literacy, and healthcare facility distribution [20].

GIS in AMR research faces challenges like data scarcity in resource-limited areas, the need for comprehensive testing, and difficulties integrating diverse datasets [14]. However, open-source GIS platforms, remote sensing data, and advanced GIS tools may offer opportunities to model AMR's spatial drivers, even in data-poor settings.

9.3.1 Common GIS Methods

Several GIS methods have been used in AMR research, including descriptive spatial analyses. Among the simplest are static maps, which effectively visualize geospatial distributions (e.g., AMR) helping policymakers identify high-prevalence areas. Beyond visualization, hotspot analysis pinpoints areas with statistically significantly clustered rates, guiding targeted interventions. Among the most common cluster detection methods are Getis-Ord G_i^* statistic [21] and LISA (Local Indicators of Spatial Association) [22]. Getis-Ord G_i^* (Eq. 9.1) assesses high, low, vs. non-significant clusters in the study area.

$$G_i^* = \frac{\sum_{j=1}^{n} w_{i,j} x_j - \bar{X} \sum_{j=1}^{n} w_{i,j}}{S \sqrt{\frac{\left[n \sum_{j=1}^{n} w^2_{i,j} - \left(\sum_{j=1}^{n} w_{i,j} \right)^2 \right]}{n-1}}} \tag{9.1}$$

In Eq. 9.1, x_j is the attribute value for feature j, $w_{i,j}$ is the spatial weight between features i and j, n is the total number of features, X^{-} is the mean value of the spatial process (i.e., AMR prevalence) and S is its standard deviation.

LISA (Eq. 9.2) identifies significant local spatial autocorrelation by measuring the similarity of neighbouring features.

$$I_i = \frac{x_i - \bar{X}}{S_i^2} \sum_{j=1, j \neq 1}^{n} w_{i,j} \left(x_i - \bar{X} \right) \tag{9.2}$$

where x_j is the attribute value for feature j, X^{-} is the mean value of the spatial process (e.g., AMR prevalence), $w_{i,j}$ is the spatial weight between features i and j, and

$$S_i^2 = \frac{\sum_{j=1, j \neq 1}^{n} \left(x_i - \bar{X} \right)^2}{n-1} \tag{9.3}$$

with n equalling the total number of features [9].

The significant clusters highlighted by both G_i^* and LISA provide researchers with a starting point to explore localized determinants. A subsequent, common analytical step is geographically weighted regression (GWR), which models spatially varying relationships between AMR and potential predictors, such as population demographics, health literacy, or access to healthcare facilities [6]. Importantly, GWR, along with other spatial analytical techniques, i.e., spatially autoregressive models (SAR) can reduce the variability of regression models on spatial data, yielding more reliable predictions [6]. Unlike traditional regression, GWR (Eq. 9.4) estimates a local parameter for every geographical unit across the study area.

$$Y_i = \beta_0 \left(u_i, v_i \right) + \sum_k \beta_k \left(u_i, v_i \right) X_{ik} + \varepsilon_i \tag{9.4}$$

In Eq.9.4 (u_i, v_i) denotes the coordinates of the ith point and $\beta_k (u_i, v_i)$ represents the value of the continuous function $\beta_k (u, v)$ at point i. Equation 9.4 can be solved using the weighted least squares approach [6] which assumes that features within a neighbourhood of point i influence the estimation of its parameters more than those further away.

GIS applications in AMR research are expanding, e.g., geospatial techniques have been used to assess the role of rurality and literacy rate in driving AMR in Malakand Division Pakistan [9]. Similarly, studies in sub-Saharan Africa and Southeast Asia have employed GIS to map resistance patterns and identify correlations with environmental and social variables, such as water quality and literacy levels [22]. These insights help tailor interventions to specific contexts, reducing the burden of AMR in vulnerable populations.

9.4 AMR in Northern Pakistan: Case Study

9.4.1 Study Area

The study area (Fig. 9.1) spans 8 districts and 28 tehsils in Pakistan's Malakand region, home to about nine million people, five major cities but mostly in rural areas (90%) and with low literacy rate (Fig. 9.2). Characterized by the rugged Himalayan foothills, the region faces harsh winters, heavy snowfall, and frequent landslides, making healthcare access challenging, especially in remote areas. Analyses were conducted at the tehsil level.

9.4.2 Study Design and Data

This study analyzed data from SGTH, a key tertiary care facility in Malakand District, collected between January and March 2021. Case histories of 548 patients,

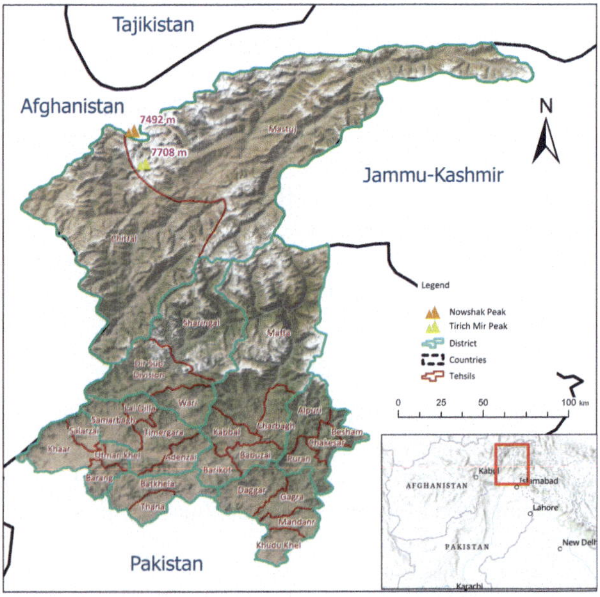

Fig. 9.1 Study area

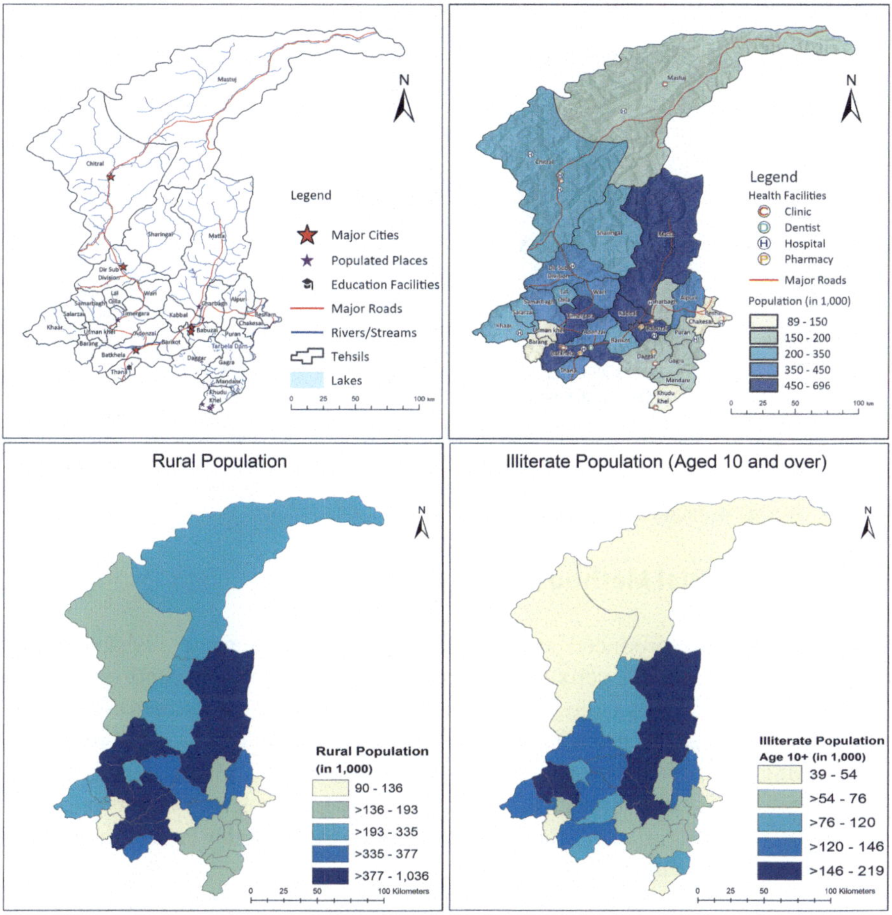

Fig. 9.2 Top Left: Major cities and populated areas; Top Right: Total population and health facilities; Bottom Left: Rural population; Bottom Right: Illiterate population

who were on antibiotics for at least 3 days, were reviewed with hospital authorization and informed consent. Culture sensitivity tests assessed resistance to cefixime, co-trimoxazole, doxycycline, and ciprofloxacin. Resistance rates were estimated using tehsil population proportions. Additional demographic data for 2023 [23], including gender, literacy, disabilities, and urban-rural distribution, was used to support spatial analysis. Figure 9.3 illustrates the entire workflow, detailing the process from data collection to spatial analysis.

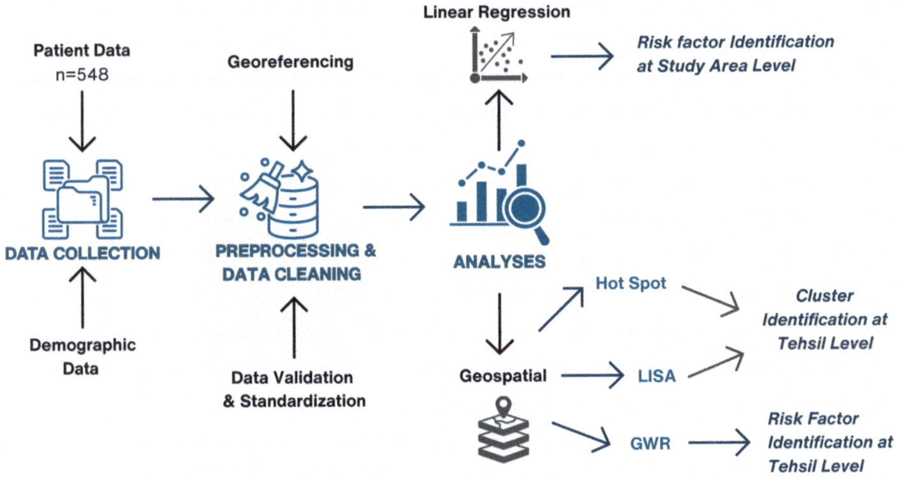

Fig. 9.3 Workflow diagram

9.4.3 Geospatial Methods & Results

Static maps were produced to visualize the distribution of resistance and resistance+sensitivity for cefixime, co-trimoxazole, doxycycline, and ciprofloxacin (Fig. 9.4). Co-trimoxazole showed the highest resistance rate (up to 92%), and when resistance and sensitivity were combined, several tehsils exhibited rates approaching 100% for all four antibiotics. The Gagra and Mastuj tehsils have a 100% rate if resistance and sensitivity are combined. For specific resistance and sensitivity rates along with Confidence Intervals (CI) of the entire study area, please refer to Fig. 9.5.

Hot spots of the resistant population (at 90%, 95%, 99% CI) and area clusters are shown in Fig. 9.6. Cefixime exhibits the largest hot spot areas with a 99% CI. A few hot spots for ciprofloxacin overlap with clusters, making them ideal initial targets for interventions.

Linear regression was applied as the global model, while GWR was used as the local model to identify significant contributing factors at the Tehsil level. For the choice of the weighting matrix in GWR [6], a golden search selection was employed to determine the optimal number of neighbours. This method first identifies the maximum and minimum nearest neighbours and then iteratively tests the AICc (Akaike Information Criterion corrected) at various distances to find the best fit. As a result, a range of 22–28 nearest neighbours was used for the GWR models. To assess local multicollinearity, the Condition Number diagnostic test was applied. A Condition Number below 30 generally indicates low multicollinearity; in our models, all Condition Numbers were below 8, confirming minimal multicollinearity.

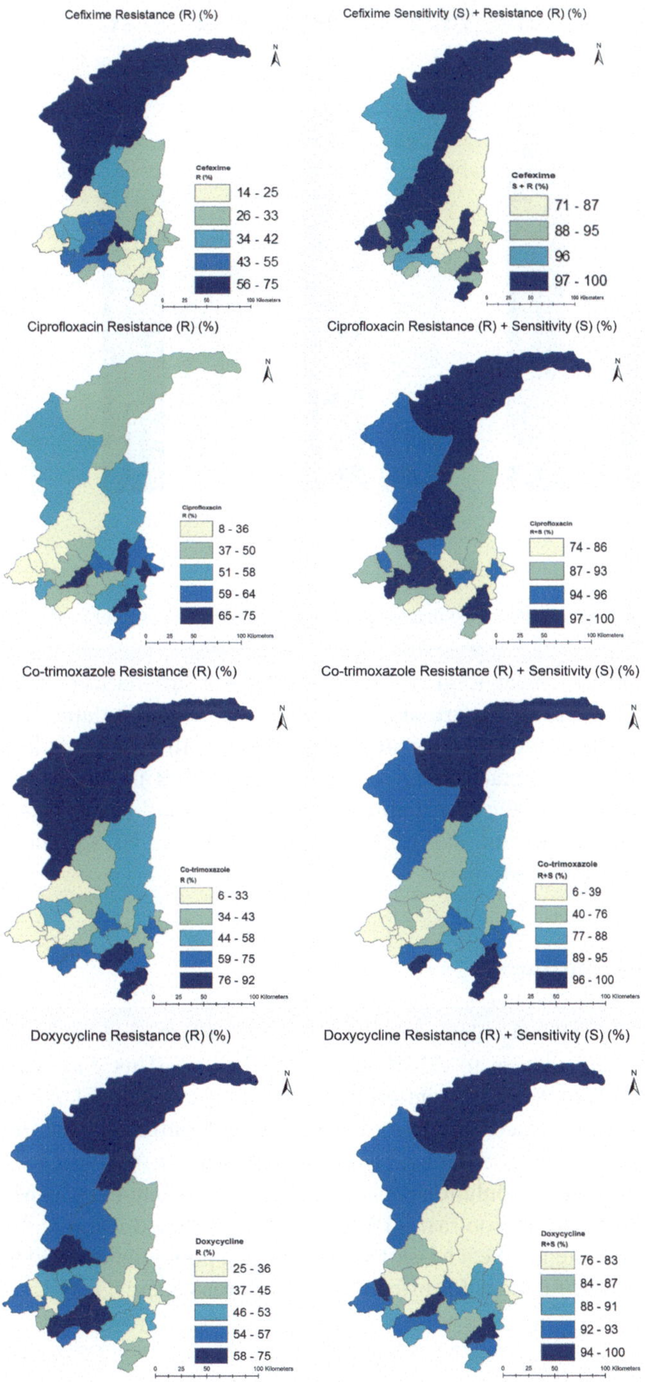

Fig. 9.4 Spatial distribution of resistance (1) and resistance+sensitivity (2) of cefixime (**a**), ciprofloxacin (**b**), co-trimoxazole (**c**), and doxycycline (**d**)

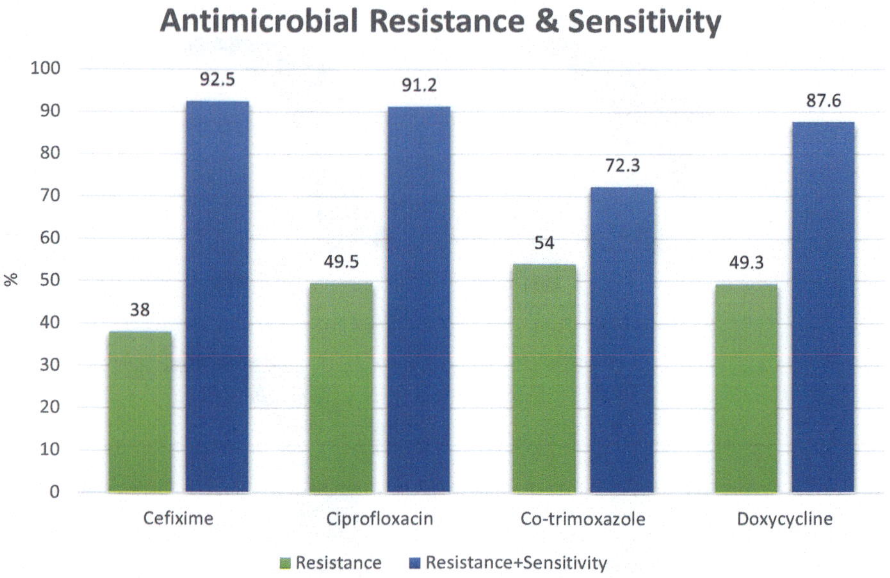

Fig. 9.5 Antibiotic specific resistance and resistance + sensitivity (combined)

The results of Linear Regression and GWR are summarized in Tables 9.1 and 9.2, respectively. Linear regression identifies the rural population as a significant factor across all antibiotics in the study area, with the illiterate population also being significant for ciprofloxacin, and co-trimoxazole. GWR provides a more localized perspective, mapping the distribution of coefficients and highlighting areas where risk factors are significant (at 90%, 95%, and 99% CI) or not significant. Figure 9.7 presents the GWR result maps.

9.4.4 Key Findings

Geospatial analysis may play a crucial role in identifying hidden hotspots, clusters, and contributing factors to AMR at the local level. This case study highlights hotspots and clusters for four antibiotics at the sub-district level. Although hotspots and clusters were detected in many tehsils for each antibiotic, the most frequently identified areas include Adenzai, Kabbal, and Wari. Linear regression identifies rural and illiterate populations as significant contributors to AMR across the Malakand Division. In contrast, GWR provides localized insights into the significance and coefficients of each risk factor, enabling policymakers and health authorities to target specific areas for effective interventions against AMR.

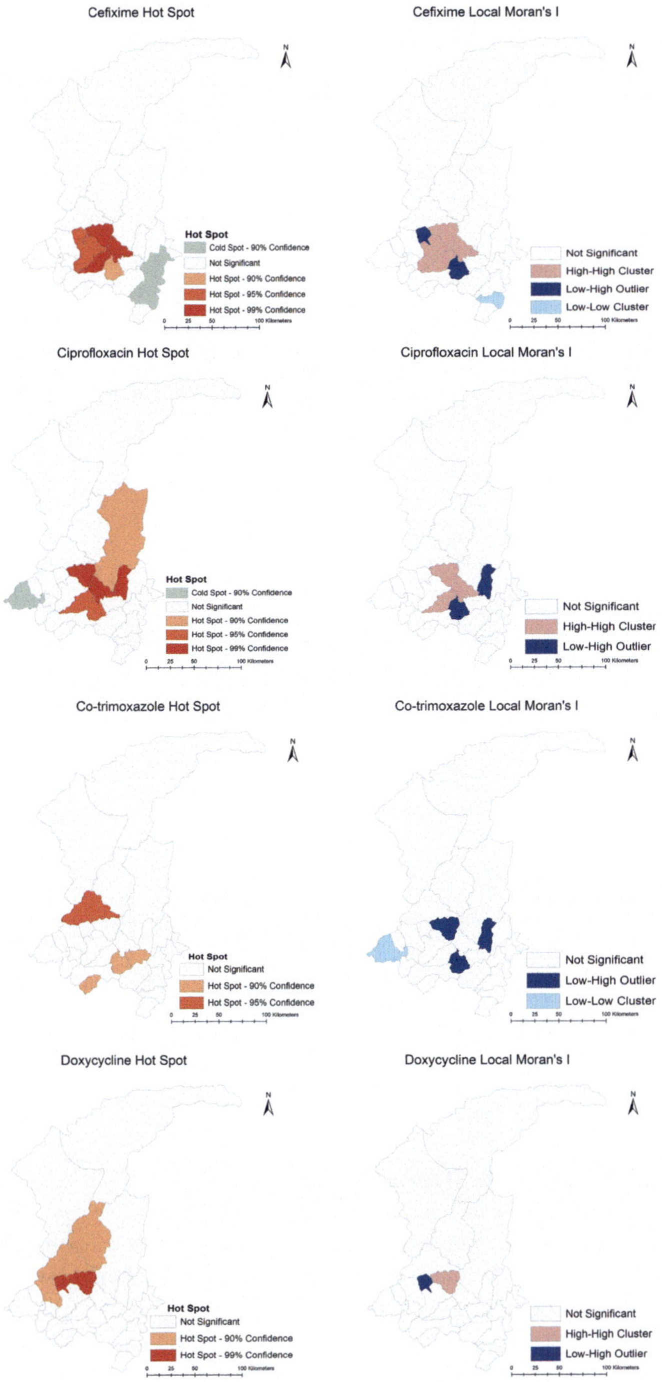

Fig. 9.6 Hot spots (left), Clusters (right)

Table 9.1 Linear regression results

Cefixime			
R Square	0.54	*Std Err*	56922.16
Adj R Sq	0.52	Sample	28
	Coef.	*Std Err*	*t Stat*
Intercept	29111.98	19576.31	1.49
Rural Pop	0.31	0.06	5.49
Co-trimoxazole			
R Square	0.49	*Std Err*	78491.31
Adj R Sq	0.45	Sample	28
	Coef.	*Std Err*	*t Stat*
Intercept	19158.01	33792.72	0.57
Rural Pop	0.74	0.37	2.00
Illiterate Pop	0.23	0.10	2.31
Ciprofloxacin			
R Square	0.64	*Std Err*	57668.93
Adj R Sq	0.61	Sample	28
	Coef.	*Std Err*	*t Stat*
Intercept	399.31	24828.1	0.02
Rural Pop	0.14	0.07	2.00
Illiterate Pop	1.04	0.27	3.83
Doxycycline			
R Square	0.88	*Std Err*	50136.57
Adj R Sq	0.87	Sample	28
	Coef.	*Std Err*	*t Stat*
Intercept	−32938.6	17242.65	−1.91
Rural Pop	0.69	0.05	13.76

Table 9.2 GWR results

	Cefixime	Ciprofloxacin	Co-trimoxazole	Doxycycline
Neighbors	22	25	25	28
Residual Squares	4.837E+10	4.8387E+10	9.068E+10	6.4002E+10
Effective Number	6.90	8.09	8.09	3.79
Sigma	47878.66	49303.35	67494.23	51412.11
R Square	0.73	0.79	0.70	0.88
Adj R Sq	0.66	0.72	0.59	0.87

9.4.5 Limitations & Strengths

Low-income countries often experience the highest AMR rates but face significant data gaps [18, 24, 25]. While socioeconomic data at the Tehsil level is unavailable, the best available demographic data for spatial analysis was used. The sample size for antibiotic resistance is limited, especially given the region's challenging terrain and resource constraints, but it provides valuable insights. This is the first study to examine AMR at the sub-district level in KPK for four antibiotics and to conduct

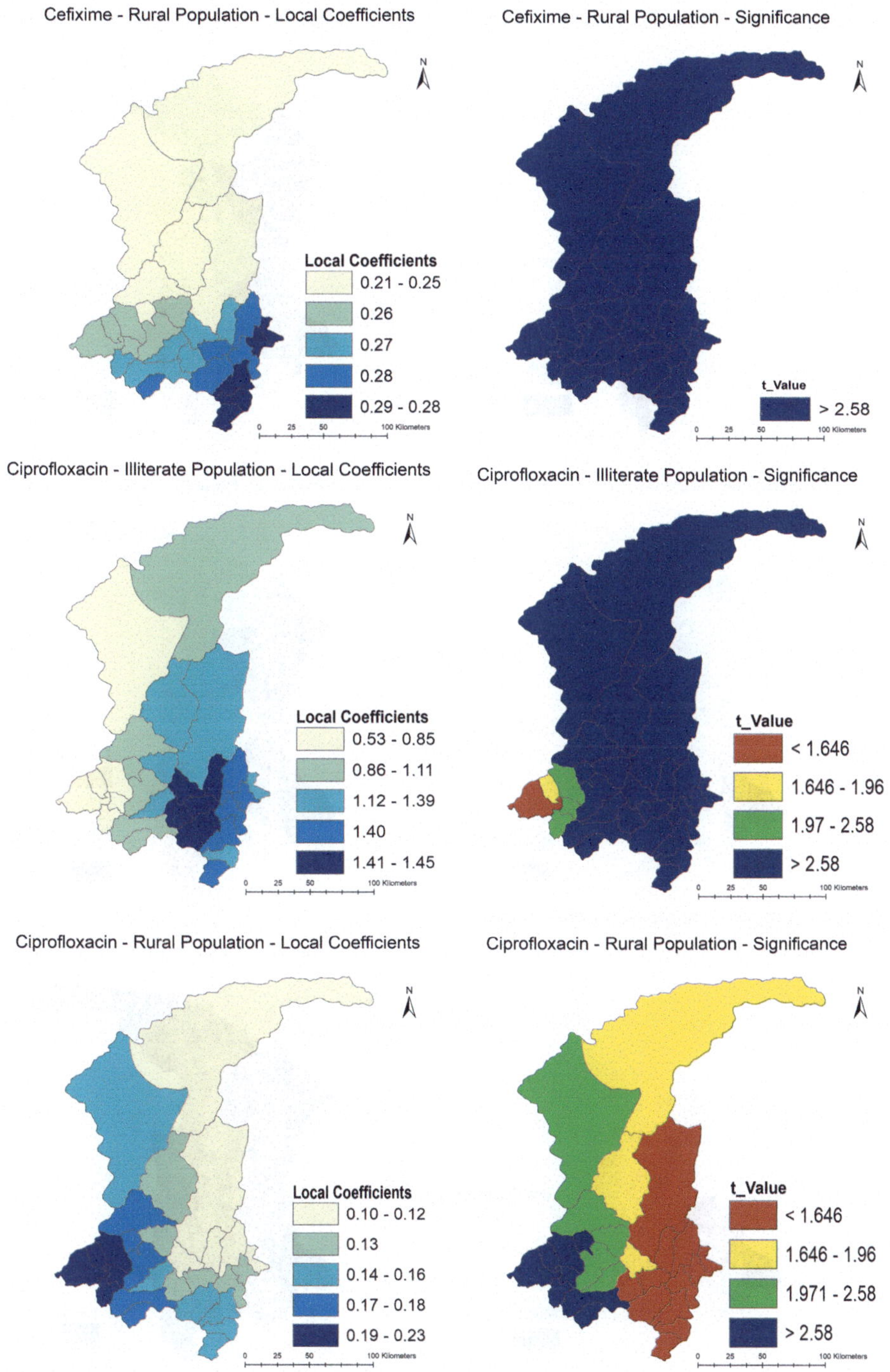

Fig. 9.7a GWR results—local coefficients & significance levels

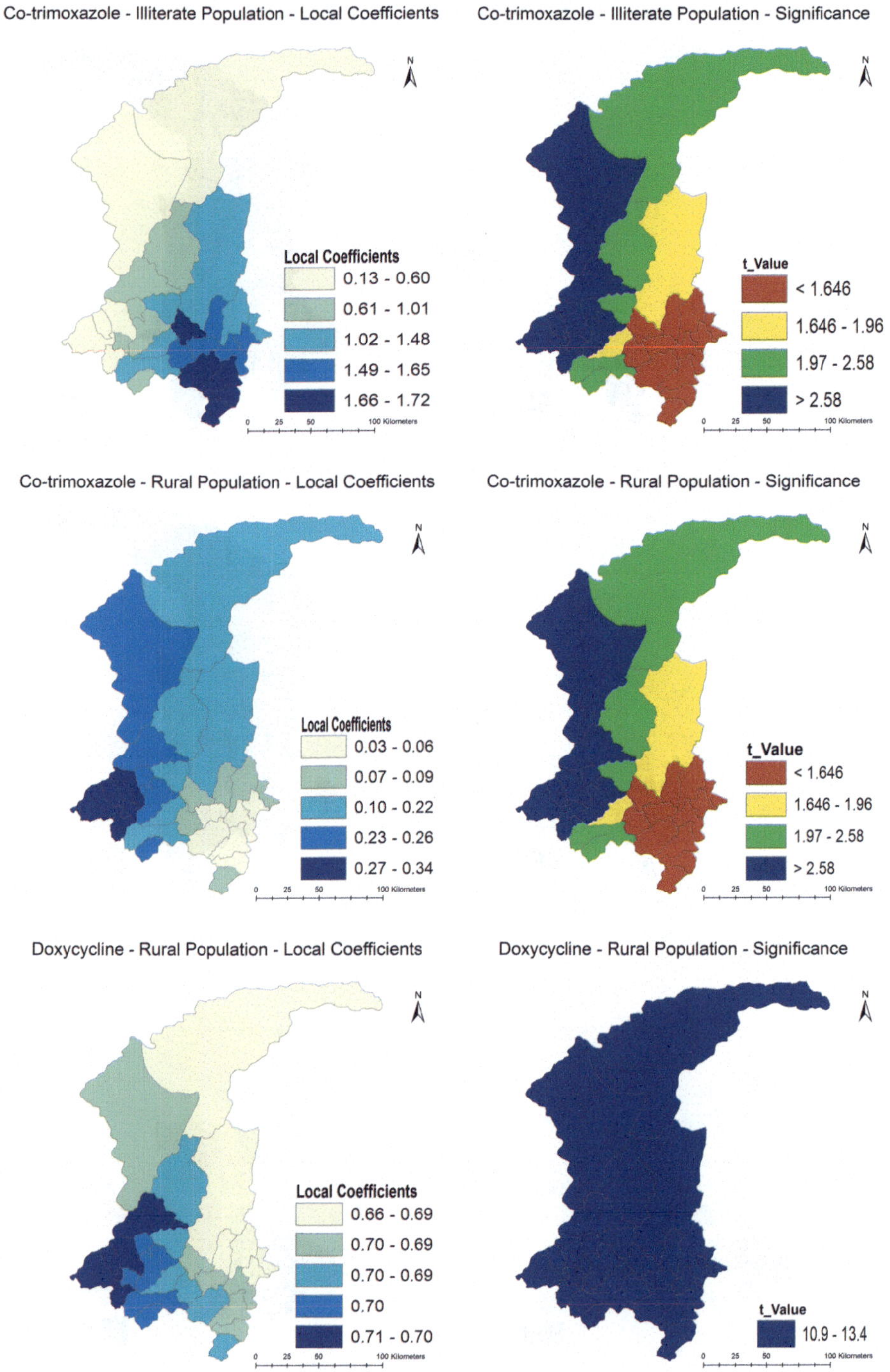

Fig. 9.7b (continued)

geospatial analyses of resistance, identifying hotspots and clusters while GWR revealed areas of local significance. Targeting high-significance areas for interventions would be more cost-effective than broader regional efforts. Additionally, preventative measures in other high-risk areas could further mitigate resistance risks.

9.5 Policy & Intervention Strategies (Conclusion)

Pakistan's policies on AMR emphasize a multi-sectoral approach guided by the National Action Plan on AMR, aligning with WHO's Global Action Plan. Despite progress, challenges persist due to limited healthcare access in remote and mountainous regions, insufficient awareness, and weak enforcement of regulatory frameworks. Geospatial tools like GIS are proving invaluable for mapping AMR hotspots in these underserved areas, enabling targeted interventions. These tools help visualize the spatial patterns of resistance, integrating environmental, healthcare, and demographic data to design effective local interventions. Scaling up from localized hotspots to regional strategies requires coordinated efforts, incorporating GIS-driven insights into national policies to ensure equitable resource allocation and sustained AMR mitigation across broader regions.

References

1. Estany-Gestal A, Salgado-Barreira A, Vazquez-Lago JM (2024) Antibiotic use and antimicrobial resistance: a global public health crisis. Antibiotics 13(9)
2. Baekkeskov E, Rubin O, Munkholm L, Zaman W (2020) Antimicrobial resistance as a global health crisis. Oxf Res Encyclopedia Politics:1–24
3. Taha BA, Ahmed NM, Talreja RK, Haider AJ, Al Mashhadany Y, Al-Jubouri Q, Huddin AB, Mokhtar MHH, Rustagi S, Kaushik A (2024) Synergizing nanomaterials and artificial intelligence in advanced optical biosensors for precision antimicrobial resistance diagnosis. ACS Synth Biol 13(6):1600–1620
4. Chaudhary V, Sable H, Kumar M, Prakash C, Sonu S (2025b) Dynamic landscape of chemiresistive breathomic nanosensors based on fifth-generation chips for complex disease diagnosis and healthcare monitoring. Appl Phys Rev 12(4)
5. Pal A, Sable H, Uniyal A, Chaudhary V (2025) Green nano-semiconductors and nanometals to avert complex phenomena of antimicrobial resistance (AMR). Curr Opin Biomed Eng 36:100626
6. Matthiessen LE, Hald T, Vigre H (2022) System mapping of antimicrobial resistance to combat a rising global health crisis. Front Public Health 10:816943
7. Singh V, Sable H, Ghalley M, Tenzin K (2024) Environmental toxicology, fate and risk assessment of emerging contaminants. In: Occurrence, distribution and toxic effects of emerging contaminants. CRC Press, pp 134–167
8. Ansari MM, Kuche K, Ghadi R, Date T, Chaudhari D, Khan R, Jain S (2022) Socioeconomic impact of antimicrobial resistance and their integrated mitigation by one health approach. In: Emerging modalities in mitigation of antimicrobial resistance. Springer, pp 135–156
9. Anselin L (1995) Local indicators of spatial association—LISA. Geogr Anal 27(2):93–115
10. Chaudhary V, Bhadola P, Kaushik A, Khalid M, Furukawa H, Khosla A (2022) Assessing temporal correlation in environmental risk factors to design efficient area-specific COVID-19 regulations: Delhi based case study. Sci Rep 12(1):12949

11. Opiyo SO, Nalunkuma R, Nanyonga SM, Mugenyi N, Kanyike AM (2024) Empowering Global AMR Research Community: interactive GIS dashboards for AMR data analysis and informed decision-making. Wellcome Open Research 9:234
12. Singh V, Kasana E, Batra J, Sable H, Saxena R (2022) Antimicrobial resistance: mechanisms, screening techniques and biosensors. J Pharm Negat Results 13:1724–1735
13. Chaudhary V, Bhadola P (2025) Artificial intelligence-powered nanosensor platforms for non-invasive breathomic diagnostics. Nanotechnol Sci Appl 18:611–641
14. Aslam B, Khurshid M, Arshad MI, Muzammil S, Rasool M, Yasmeen N, Shah T, Chaudhry TH, Rasool MH, Shahid A (2021) Antibiotic resistance: one health one world outlook. Front Cell Infect Microbiol 11:771510
15. Arnold KE, Laing G, McMahon BJ, Fanning S, Stekel DJ, Pahl O, Coyne L, Latham SM, McIntyre KM (2024) The need for One Health systems-thinking approaches to understand multiscale dissemination of antimicrobial resistance. Lancet Planet Heath 8(2):e124–e133
16. Asghar A, Khalid A, Baqar Z, Hussain N, Saleem MZ, Sairash, Rizwan K (2024) An insights into emerging trends to control the threats of antimicrobial resistance (AMR): an address to public health risks. Arch Microbiol 206(2):72
17. Zahir S, Khan K, Sardar N, Jahan S, Ali MM, Khan A, Khattak J, Mazhar S, Shah J (2024) Insights into standard precaution knowledge and adherence among healthcare workers: evidence from tertiary care hospitals in Peshawar, Pakistan: standard precautions and healthcare workers. Pak J Health Sci:19–24
18. Chaudhary V, Lucky L, Sable H, Bhalla N (2025a) Interdisciplinary approach to monkeypox prevention: integrating nanobiosensors, nanovaccines, artificial intelligence, visual arts, and social sciences. Small Struct 6:2400647
19. Ghani S, Khan N, Sable H, Yao F, Shafiq M (2025) Computational techniques for enhancing PK/PD modeling and simulation and ADMET prediction. In: Computational methods in medicinal chemistry, pharmacology, and toxicology. Elsevier, pp 153–174
20. Nykiforuk CI, Flaman LM (2011) Geographic information systems (GIS) for health promotion and public health: a review. Health Promot Pract 12(1):63–73
21. Getis A, Ord JK (1992) The analysis of spatial association by use of distance statistics. Geogr Anal 24(3):189–206
22. Lewnard JA, Lo NC, Arinaminpathy N, Frost I, Laxminarayan R (2020) Childhood vaccines and antibiotic use in low-and middle-income countries. Nature 581(7806):94–99
23. Rahman R, Sheehan D, Javed A, Ahmed SH, Shafique K, Kanwal U, Afridi MI, Tamizuddin Nizami A, Rasool G, Taj R (2024). The National Psychiatric Morbidity Survey of Pakistan (2022): prevalence, socio-demographic and disability correlates. medRxiv 2024.2007.2008.24310056
24. Chaudhary V, Gaur P, Rustagi S (2024) Sensors, society, and sustainability. Sustain Mater Technol 40:e00952
25. Murray CJ, Ikuta KS, Sharara F, Swetschinski L, Aguilar GR, Gray A, Han C, Bisignano C, Rao P, Wool E (2022) Global burden of bacterial antimicrobial resistance in 2019: a systematic analysis. Lancet 399(10325):629–655

Antibiotic Abuse Surveillance: Future Prospects

10

Oyindamola John Samson,
Stephen Olaosebikan Makanjuola,
Abosede Olubunmi Obadina, Ayush Madan,
Moses Sunday Afariogun, and Ismail Babatunde Onajobi

10.1 Introduction

The widespread misuse and overuse of antibiotics have become a significant driver of antimicrobial resistance (AMR), a critical global health challenge threatening the efficacy of modern medicine. Antibiotic abuse, often characterized by self-medication, over-prescription, and the use of antibiotics in agriculture and aquaculture, exacerbates the emergence and spread of resistant pathogens [14]. AMR not only leads to increased morbidity and mortality but also imposes substantial economic burdens on healthcare systems worldwide. This crisis requires multifaceted

O. J. Samson (✉)
Department of Microbiology, Faculty of Science, Olabisi Onabanjo University, Ago-Iwoye, Nigeria

Department of Microbiology and Biotechnology, Faculty of Natural Sciences, Ajayi Crowther University, Oyo, Nigeria

S. O. Makanjuola
Department of Medical Laboratory Science, Faculty of Allied Health Science, Elizade University, Ilara-Mokin, Nigeria

A. O. Obadina
Department of Public Health, College of Allied Health Science, McPherson University, Seriki Sotayo, Nigeria

A. Madan
Department of Biotechnology, School of Research and Technology, People's University, Bhopal, Madhya Pradesh, India

M. S. Afariogun
Department of Cell Biology and Genetics, University of Lagos, Akoka, Nigeria

I. B. Onajobi
Department of Microbiology, Faculty of Science, Olabisi Onabanjo University, Ago-Iwoye, Nigeria

V. Chaudhary, N. Bhalla (eds.), *Biosensors for Tackling Antimicrobial Resistance (AMR)*, https://doi.org/10.1007/978-981-95-9151-0_10

approaches, among which the surveillance of antibiotic usage and resistance patterns plays a pivotal role in informing effective interventions and policies [26].

Traditional surveillance systems, while valuable, often face limitations that hinder their efficiency in capturing real-time data. These systems rely heavily on manual reporting and laboratory analyses, which are time-consuming and resource-intensive [19]. Furthermore, in low- and middle-income countries, where the burden of AMR is often higher, surveillance infrastructure is often inadequate or absent. As a result, gaps in data availability and accuracy impede efforts to combat antibiotic abuse effectively. The need for innovative solutions to overcome these challenges is more pressing than ever [37].

Biosensors have emerged as a promising technological innovation in the realm of antibiotic abuse surveillance. These devices offer rapid, sensitive, and cost-effective means to detect and monitor antibiotics and resistant pathogens across various settings, including clinical, agricultural, and environmental domains [3]. Advancements in nanotechnology, microfluidics, and artificial intelligence, biosensors can transform the way antibiotic usage and resistance patterns are tracked, enabling real-time data acquisition and analysis. Their potential to bridge gaps in traditional surveillance systems makes them a cornerstone of future strategies to tackle AMR [44].

The integration of biosensors with digital health platforms further enhances their capabilities, providing a seamless flow of information from detection to decision-making. Internet of Things (IoT) devices and cloud computing technologies enable biosensors to operate at scale, facilitating large-scale data collection and processing [52]. Such integration supports proactive interventions, informed policymaking, and the efficient allocation of resources, particularly in regions with limited healthcare infrastructure. The convergence of biosensors and digital health represents a paradigm shift in antibiotic stewardship and AMR management [17].

The future prospects of antibiotic abuse surveillance, focusing on the transformative role of biosensors. It begins by examining the challenges and limitations of current surveillance methods, followed by a detailed discussion on technological advancements in biosensor design and application [32]. Case studies illustrating successful implementations and addresses potential barriers to widespread adoption are also been highlighted. The integration of biosensors with digital health and offering recommendations for future directions, this review explains the pivotal role of innovation in combating antibiotic abuse and mitigating the AMR crisis.

10.2 Current Challenges in Antibiotic Abuse Surveillance

The fight against antimicrobial resistance (AMR) is critically dependent on effective surveillance systems to monitor antibiotic use and resistance patterns. However, existing surveillance approaches face several challenges that limit their efficacy. Traditional surveillance methods rely on manual data collection, laboratory-based analyses, and fragmented reporting systems, which are often characterized by delays in data reporting and analysis [48]. These delays hinder timely interventions and policy formulation, allowing the unchecked progression of antibiotic abuse and resistance. Furthermore, the reliance on centralized laboratory facilities restricts real-time tracking, particularly in rural or resource-limited regions [12].

One of the significant barriers to effective antibiotic abuse surveillance is inadequate coverage, especially in low-resource settings. Many developing nations lack the necessary infrastructure, trained personnel, and financial resources to establish robust surveillance frameworks. In such contexts, underreporting and incomplete data are common, leading to a skewed understanding of antibiotic use and resistance trends. The disparity in surveillance capabilities between high-income and low-income regions exacerbates global inequities in addressing AMR [28].

Compounding these issues is the presence of knowledge gaps in antibiotic use patterns across different sectors. Surveillance systems often focus predominantly on clinical settings, neglecting the agricultural and environmental sectors, where antibiotics are extensively used and misused. The lack of integrated surveillance systems that encompass all these sectors contributes to an incomplete understanding of the drivers of AMR. For instance, antibiotics used in livestock production can enter the environment through wastewater, creating hotspots for resistance gene proliferation—a phenomenon that remains underreported due to sectoral silos [31].

Efforts to address these challenges must consider the heterogeneity in antibiotic usage practices and resistance dynamics across regions and sectors. A comprehensive and integrated surveillance approach is necessary to capture real-time, accurate data that reflects the multidimensional nature of antibiotic abuse (Table 10.1). This would not only enhance the efficacy of AMR interventions but also inform global strategies for antibiotic stewardship [24].

10.3 Role of Biosensors in Antibiotic Abuse Surveillance

Biosensors are analytical devices that combine a biological sensing element with a physicochemical transducer to detect target substances. In the context of antibiotic abuse surveillance, biosensors are designed to identify antibiotics, resistant pathogens, or resistance genes in various samples, including clinical specimens, agricultural products, and environmental samples. These devices typically consist of three main components: a bioreceptor, such as enzymes, antibodies, or nucleic acids; a transducer that converts the biological interaction into a measurable signal; and a signal processing unit that displays the results. The versatility and adaptability of biosensors make them highly suitable for monitoring antibiotic use and resistance trends [13].

One of the primary advantages of biosensors over conventional surveillance tools is their ability to provide rapid detection. Unlike traditional methods, which often require time-consuming laboratory analyses, biosensors can deliver results within minutes or hours. This speed is critical for real-time monitoring, enabling healthcare providers and policymakers to respond promptly to emerging patterns of antibiotic misuse and resistance. For instance, point-of-care biosensors in clinical settings can quickly detect resistant pathogens, facilitating timely treatment decisions and reducing the spread of resistance [20].

Table 10.1 Challenges in antibiotic abuse surveillance

Challenge	Description	Impact	Examples	References
Delayed Data Reporting	Reliance on manual processes leads to slow data collection and reporting	Hinders timely interventions and policy responses	Delayed recognition of resistance outbreaks in hospitals	Lee et al. [27]
Inadequate Coverage	Lack of infrastructure in low-resource settings limits surveillance reach	Creates data gaps and inequities in AMR understanding	Limited surveillance in rural regions of sub-Saharan Africa	Rony et al. [42]
Sectoral Knowledge Gaps	Focus on clinical settings neglects agricultural and environmental sectors	Fails to capture holistic antibiotic use and resistance	Antibiotics in livestock waste leading to environmental resistance hotspots	Kunhikannan et al. [25]
Resource Constraints	Insufficient funding, personnel, and technology in developing countries	Reduces the scope and quality of surveillance efforts	Underfunded AMR programs in Southeast Asia	Shrestha et al. [46]
Fragmented Reporting Systems	Lack of integration among different data sources and sectors	Prevents comprehensive data analysis and action	Separate reporting systems for human health and agriculture in many regions	Prickett et al. [38]

Biosensors also offer unparalleled sensitivity and specificity in detecting antibiotic residues or resistance markers. The integration of advanced technologies, such as nanomaterials and engineered bioreceptors, enhances their ability to detect minute concentrations of targets with high accuracy. This precision minimizes false positives and false negatives, ensuring reliable.

surveillance data. In agricultural contexts, biosensors can accurately monitor antibiotic residues in livestock or crops, supporting better regulatory compliance and reducing the environmental impact of antibiotic use [54].

Another notable advantage of biosensors is their cost-effectiveness. Traditional surveillance methods often involve expensive equipment, extensive manpower, and centralized facilities, which can be prohibitive in low-resource settings. Biosensors, on the other hand, are often portable, user-friendly, and require minimal training, making them accessible to a broader range of users. Their affordability and scalability enable widespread adoption, particularly in regions where AMR surveillance infrastructure is underdeveloped [53].

The role of biosensors in antibiotic surveillance (Fig. 10.1), highlighting three key components: **Inputs** (clinical, agricultural, and environmental samples), **Biosensor Components** (bioreceptor, transducer, and signal processor for detecting antibiotics or resistance), and **Outputs** (real-time detection, policymaking data, and insights for various sectors). Arrows connect these elements, showcasing a systematic workflow for effective monitoring and decision-making.

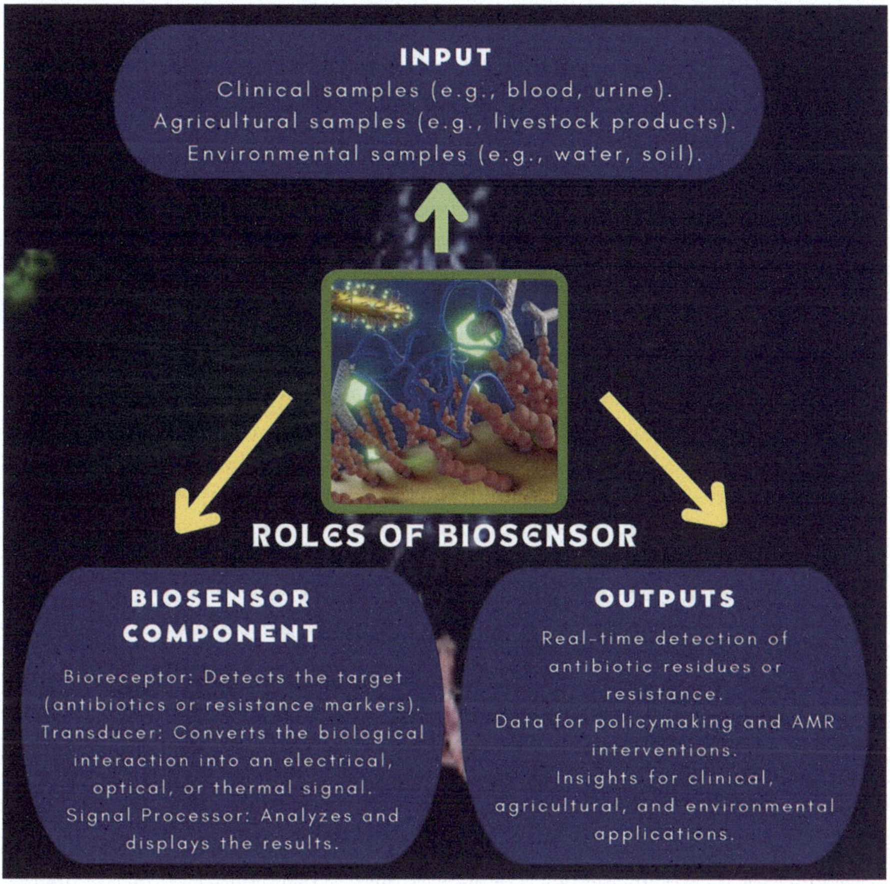

Fig. 10.1 Role of biosensors in antibiotic surveillance

10.4 Technological Innovations in Biosensor Design

The field of biosensor technology has seen significant advancements in recent years, driven by the integration of cutting-edge innovations. Nanotechnology has revolutionized biosensor design by enabling the development of nanoscale materials that enhance sensitivity and specificity. Nanomaterials such as nanoparticles, carbon nanotubes, and graphene are widely used as bioreceptor supports or signal enhancers [39]. Their high surface area, excellent conductivity, and unique optical properties enable the detection of even trace amounts of antibiotics or resistance markers, significantly improving the efficiency of biosensors. Microfluidics complements these advancements by miniaturizing the detection system into compact, efficient devices. Microfluidic platforms allow precise sample handling and integration of multiple detection steps within a single chip, reducing analysis time and reagent use [34].

Artificial intelligence (AI) and machine learning (ML) are increasingly being incorporated into biosensor technology to enhance data processing capabilities. AI algorithms analyze complex datasets generated by biosensors, identifying patterns and correlations that would otherwise be challenging to detect manually [11]. Machine learning models can be trained to predict antibiotic resistance trends based on biosensor data, enabling proactive interventions. Additionally, AI-driven image analysis is used in optical biosensors to interpret colorimetric or fluorescence signals with higher accuracy [15]. The combination of biosensors with AI and ML has led to the development of smart surveillance systems capable of real-time monitoring and decision-making [6, 55].

The development of portable and user-friendly biosensors has been a game-changer in expanding the accessibility of these devices. The outcome of advancing in materials science and electronics, researchers have created biosensors that are compact, lightweight, and easy to operate. These portable devices are particularly valuable in resource-limited settings, where traditional laboratory facilities are unavailable. Point-of-care biosensors, designed for use by non-specialists, enable on-site testing in clinical, agricultural, and environmental contexts. Such innovations democratize access to AMR surveillance, empowering a wider range of stakeholders to participate in combating antibiotic abuse [23, 49].

Integration of these technologies has also improved the scalability of biosensor applications. Devices that combine nanotechnology, microfluidics, AI, and portability are now being produced at lower costs, facilitating their adoption on a larger scale. For example, portable biosensors embedded with AI-driven data analytics can be deployed in remote areas, enabling comprehensive and inclusive surveillance. Furthermore, such innovations support decentralized monitoring systems, reducing the reliance on centralized laboratories and enhancing the resilience of AMR strategies [5].

Despite these advancements, challenges such as standardization, regulatory approval, and commercialization remain. Addressing these issues will require coordinated efforts among researchers, industry stakeholders, and policymakers. Continued investment in R&D and international collaborations are essential to fully harness the potential of these technological innovations in biosensor design (Table 10.2).

10.5 Applications of Biosensors in Surveillance

Biosensors have emerged as transformative tools in monitoring antibiotic use and resistance across various sectors. In clinical settings, these devices play a critical role in ensuring judicious antibiotic prescription and improving patient compliance. Biosensors can provide real-time data on the presence of antibiotic-resistant pathogens in patients, enabling healthcare providers to tailor treatments more effectively. Additionally, wearable biosensors can monitor drug levels in a patient's bloodstream, ensuring that prescribed antibiotics are taken correctly and within therapeutic ranges, thereby reducing the likelihood of resistance development [29].

Table 10.2 Technological innovations in biosensor design

Innovation	Description	Advantages	Applications	References
Nanotechnology	Use of nanoscale materials (e.g., nanoparticles, graphene) to enhance sensitivity and specificity	Detection of trace antibiotics or resistance markers; increased signal amplification	Clinical diagnostics, residue detection in food and water	Ramesh et al. [39]
Microfluidics	Miniaturized systems for precise sample handling and analysis	Reduces sample volume, analysis time, and costs; allows multiplex detection	Portable lab-on-a-chip devices for field applications	Chamoli and Kumar [5]
Artificial Intelligence (AI)	Algorithms analyze biosensor data to identify trends and correlations	Improves accuracy, enables real-time decision-making, and predicts resistance	AI-driven image analysis for optical biosensors; trend forecasting in AMR	Flynn and Chang [15]
Machine Learning (ML)	Models trained to process complex biosensor datasets	Enhances data processing, enables predictive analytics	Training ML models to identify emerging resistance patterns	Zhang et al. [55]
Portable Biosensors	Compact, user-friendly devices for on-site testing	Increases accessibility, reduces dependence on centralized labs	Point-of-care testing in rural areas, field monitoring in agriculture	Pal et al. [36]

In the agricultural sector, biosensors are invaluable for tracking antibiotic usage in livestock, a significant contributor to antimicrobial resistance (AMR). These devices can detect antibiotic residues in animal feed, milk, and meat, ensuring that farmers adhere to regulatory limits. By identifying misuse or overuse of antibiotics in animal husbandry, biosensors help mitigate the transmission of resistance genes from animals to humans. This surveillance also supports the development of antibiotic stewardship programs tailored to agricultural practices [10, 35].

Environmental monitoring is another critical application of biosensors, focusing on detecting antibiotic residues in soil and water. Antibiotics used in clinical and agricultural settings often enter the environment through wastewater, manure, or runoff, creating resistance hotspots. Biosensors equipped with advanced detection capabilities can identify trace amounts of these residues, facilitating timely interventions to prevent ecological damage. Such monitoring also informs policies on wastewater management and environmental protection [7, 18].

The integration of biosensors across these sectors promotes a "One Health" approach to tackling AMR. This holistic perspective recognizes the interconnectedness of human, animal, and environmental health. Biosensors, by enabling comprehensive and real-time surveillance, bridge data gaps between sectors, ensuring that interventions are both informed and impactful. They provide the scientific basis for coordinated global efforts to address antibiotic misuse and its cascading consequences [9, 43, 47].

Moving forward, the scalability and accessibility of biosensors will be pivotal in maximizing their impact. Advances in portable biosensor technology, combined with artificial intelligence for data interpretation, can expand their reach to resource-limited settings. Whether in rural clinics, small-scale farms, or remote environmental sites, biosensors promise to revolutionize AMR surveillance and create a more sustainable future [45].

10.6 Integration with Digital Health Platforms

The integration of biosensors with digital health platforms represents a major advancement in antibiotic surveillance. The Internet of Things (IoT) and cloud computing are pivotal in this transformation. IoT-enabled biosensors can collect data in real-time and transmit it wirelessly to cloud-based platforms for analysis and storage. This seamless connection allows for continuous monitoring across diverse settings, including hospitals, farms, and remote environmental sites. Cloud computing provides the computational power to process vast amounts of biosensor data, enabling the identification of trends, anomalies, and emerging antibiotic resistance hotspots [50].

Real-time data collection through these integrated systems offers significant advantages. Continuous monitoring ensures timely detection of resistance patterns or antibiotic misuse, enabling immediate interventions to prevent escalation. Additionally, the ability to analyze data on a large scale allows stakeholders to visualize regional and global trends in antimicrobial resistance. This capacity supports data-driven decision-making, enhancing the precision of policy recommendations and public health strategies. For example, digital health platforms can alert healthcare providers to emerging resistance in their area, prompting stricter prescription protocols or targeted patient education campaigns [30].

Successful integrations of biosensors with digital health platforms highlight their potential. In clinical settings, biosensors connected to electronic health records (EHRs) can provide instant updates on patient drug levels and adherence, improving treatment outcomes. Similarly, in agriculture, IoT-enabled biosensors can monitor antibiotic residues in real-time, transmitting the data to centralized platforms that guide regulatory enforcement or advisory services for farmers. Environmental monitoring platforms equipped with biosensor networks can deliver actionable insights on contamination levels, supporting sustainable environmental management [52].

The integration of digital health platforms with biosensors for antibiotic surveillance (Fig. 10.2). It outlines four stages: **Data Collection** (IoT-enabled biosensors detect antibiotics or resistance markers), **Data Transmission** (real-time wireless data transfer to cloud platforms), **Data Processing** (cloud computing analyzes trends, anomalies, and resistance patterns), and **Data Utilization** (insights inform

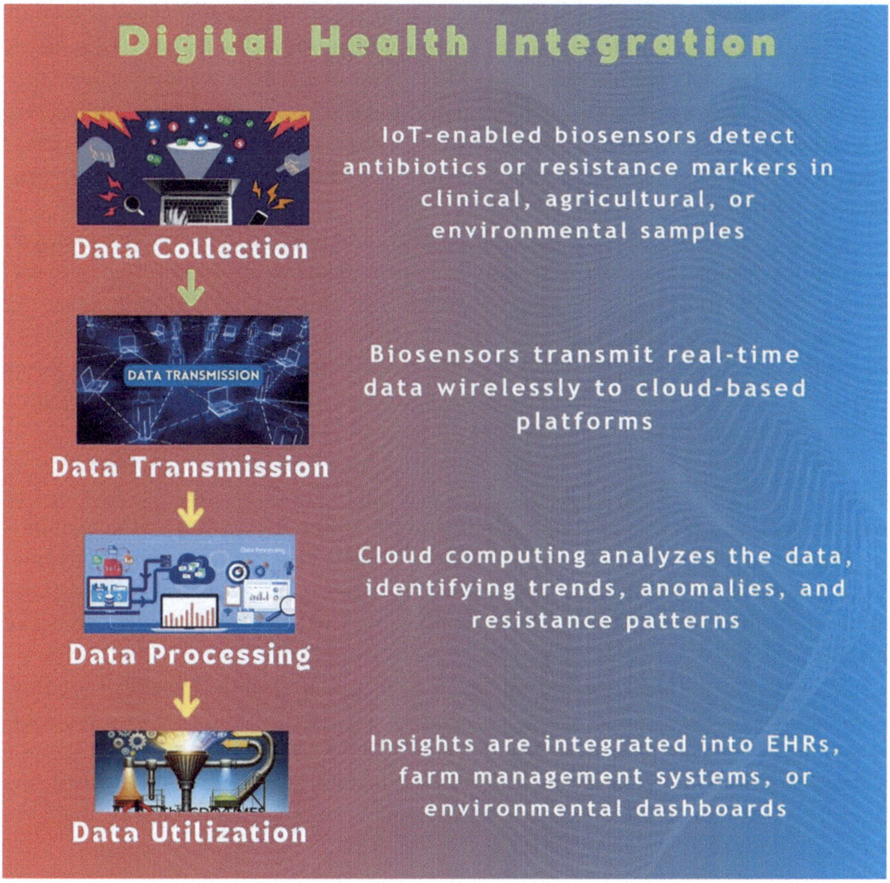

Fig. 10.2 Digital health integration workflow

electronic health records (EHRs), farm management, or environmental dashboards). The systematic flow highlights how digital tools enhance antibiotic stewardship and antimicrobial resistance (AMR) management.

10.7 Case Studies of Biosensor Implementation in Different Regions

The implementation of biosensors in various regions highlights their transformative impact on antibiotic stewardship and antimicrobial resistance (AMR) reduction. These case studies showcase how biosensor technology can bridge gaps in monitoring and facilitate targeted interventions. From clinical applications in high-resource settings to environmental monitoring in developing countries, the adaptability of biosensors is evident [4].

In Europe, biosensors have been integrated into hospital systems to monitor antibiotic levels in patients undergoing treatment. For example, in the UK, biosensors linked to electronic health records (EHRs) track patient compliance and drug metabolism, ensuring antibiotics are used optimally. This approach has significantly reduced incidences of under-dosing or over-dosing, minimizing the risk of resistance development. The data generated also informs hospital-wide stewardship programs, leading to more judicious use of antibiotics [1, 16].

In India, a country grappling with high rates of AMR, biosensors are employed to monitor antibiotic residues in livestock. Pilot projects in rural farming communities use portable biosensors to detect antibiotics in animal feed and milk, ensuring compliance with regulatory limits. This initiative has empowered farmers with actionable insights, reducing misuse and preventing the spread of resistance genes from animals to humans. Such programs also strengthen export compliance for agricultural products, boosting economic opportunities [51].

Environmental monitoring in sub-Saharan Africa demonstrates another crucial application of biosensors. In Kenya, biosensor networks have been established in water bodies near pharmaceutical manufacturing zones. These systems detect antibiotic residues in real-time, enabling rapid interventions to mitigate environmental contamination. By identifying hotspots of resistance gene dissemination, these efforts contribute to a broader understanding of AMR dynamics in low-resource settings [33].

These examples underline the importance of region-specific biosensor applications tailored to local challenges as shown in Table 10.3. While high-resource settings benefit from advanced integrations like IoT and AI, resource-limited regions leverage portable and cost-effective biosensor technologies. Across the board, the impact is clear—biosensors enhance surveillance, promote accountability, and support global efforts to combat AMR [8].

10.8 Challenges and Limitations Leading in Barriers to Biosensor Adoption

Despite the immense potential of biosensors in antibiotic surveillance, several challenges hinder their widespread adoption, particularly in low-resource settings. The high initial costs of biosensor technologies and the requirement for skilled personnel to operate and maintain them are significant barriers. For many healthcare facilities, agricultural operations, and environmental monitoring programs in developing regions, these costs remain prohibitive. Additionally, access to essential components such as reagents and advanced electronics is often limited, further restricting the use of biosensors in resource-constrained settings [21].

Regulatory and ethical considerations present another major challenge. The deployment of biosensors often involves the collection and transmission of sensitive data, raising concerns about privacy and data security. Regulatory frameworks governing biosensor applications vary significantly across regions, creating inconsistencies in adoption and implementation. Establishing universal standards for data

Table 10.3 Case studies on biosensor implementation

Region	Application	Technology used	Impact on Stewardship/ AMR	References
UK (Europe)	Monitoring antibiotic levels in patients	Biosensors integrated with EHRs	Reduced improper dosing, improved compliance, and informed hospital-wide stewardship	Garzón et al. [16]
India (Asia)	Tracking antibiotic residues in livestock	Portable biosensors for milk and feed	Reduced misuse in animal husbandry and compliance with export standards	Upadhyay and Singh [51]
Kenya (Africa)	Environmental monitoring of water bodies	Biosensor networks in water systems	Identified contamination hotspots, supported timely interventions, and mitigated resistance gene spread	Mutunga et al. [33]
USA (North America)	Rapid detection of resistance genes	AI-enhanced biosensors	Real-time tracking of resistance patterns, supporting data-driven public health policies	Banerjee and Patel [2]
China (Asia)	Industrial-scale monitoring in agriculture	IoT-enabled biosensors in aquaculture	Reduced overuse in fish farming, improved sustainability, and enhanced export compliance	Huang and Khabusi [22]

handling and device validation is critical to ensuring trust and compliance among users and stakeholders [3].

Scalability is a persistent issue with biosensor technologies. While biosensors have demonstrated efficacy in pilot programs, scaling up these systems to cover larger populations or regions can be technically and logistically complex. Challenges include integrating biosensors with existing infrastructures, maintaining their functionality in diverse environmental conditions, and ensuring the availability of support systems such as IoT networks and cloud computing [40].

Standardization also poses a significant limitation. The lack of universally accepted protocols for biosensor design, calibration, and data interpretation hinders cross-sectoral collaboration and interoperability. This inconsistency can lead to variations in performance, reduced reliability, and difficulties in comparing data across different systems or regions. Addressing standardization is essential for the global deployment of biosensors in antibiotic surveillance [41].

10.9 Conclusion

Biosensors represent a transformative tool in the fight against antibiotic misuse and antimicrobial resistance (AMR), offering innovative solutions for surveillance across clinical, agricultural, and environmental sectors. Their ability to deliver rapid, accurate, and cost-effective data has revolutionized traditional monitoring methods, enabled timely interventions and promoted more sustainable antibiotic stewardship practices. The integration of digital health platforms and leveraging advances in nanotechnology, artificial intelligence, and microfluidics, biosensors provide unprecedented opportunities for real-time surveillance and large-scale data analysis. However, maximizing their potential requires addressing challenges such as cost barriers, scalability, and standardization, particularly in low-resource settings where AMR burdens are often highest. Establishing global frameworks for the ethical and regulatory deployment of biosensors will be crucial to ensuring widespread adoption and equitable access. Aligning these technological advancements with global AMR strategies, such as the "One Health" approach, can create a comprehensive system for combating resistance, connecting human, animal, and environmental health. Biosensors not only enhance our ability to monitor and mitigate AMR but also contribute to the broader goals of sustainable development and public health. As we move forward, collaborative efforts from researchers, policymakers, and industry leaders will be essential to bridging gaps, fostering innovation, and ensuring that biosensors play a central role in the global response to antibiotic abuse. In this era of advancing technology, biosensors hold the promise of transforming AMR surveillance and safeguarding the efficacy of antibiotics for future generations.

References

1. Avershina E, Shapovalova V, Shipulin G (2021) Fighting antibiotic resistance in hospital-acquired infections: current state and emerging technologies in disease prevention, diagnostics and therapy. Front Microbiol 12:707330. https://doi.org/10.3389/fmicb.2021.707330
2. Banerjee R, Patel R (2023) Molecular diagnostics for genotypic detection of antibiotic resistance: current landscape and future directions. JAC-Antimicrobial Resistance 5(1):dlad018. https://doi.org/10.1093/jacamr/dlad018
3. Bhatia D, Paul S, Acharjee T, Ramachairy SS (2024) Biosensors and their widespread impact on human health. Sensors Int 5:100257. https://doi.org/10.1016/j.sintl.2023.100257
4. Branda F, Scarpa F (2024) Implications of artificial intelligence in addressing antimicrobial resistance: innovations, global challenges, and healthcare's future. Antibiotics 13(6):502. https://doi.org/10.3390/antibiotics13060502
5. Chamoli S, Kumar P (2024) Current challenges and future prospects of next-generation microfluidics. In: Next-generation smart biosensing. Academic, pp 307–315. https://doi.org/10.1016/B978-0-323-98805-6.00009-9
6. Chaudhary V, Gaur P, Rustagi S (2024) Sensors, society, and sustainability. Sustain Mater Technol 40:e00952
7. Chaudhary V, Lucky L, Sable H, Bhalla N (2025) Interdisciplinary approach to Monkeypox prevention: integrating nanobiosensors, nanovaccines, artificial intelligence, visual arts, and social sciences. Small Struct 6:2400647
8. Chugh P, Soni S, Chahar M, Ghanghas N, Mohan H (2025) Genosensors in healthcare. In: Fundamentals of biosensors in healthcare. Academic, pp 589–610. https://doi.org/10.1016/B978-0-443-21658-9.02004-0
9. Coman LI, Ianculescu M, Paraschiv EA, Alexandru A, Bădărău IA (2024) Smart solutions for diet-related disease management: connected care, remote health monitoring systems, and integrated insights for advanced evaluation. Appl Sci 14(6):2351. https://doi.org/10.3390/app14062351

10. Damathia B, Pathania D, Jha A, Sable H, Singh P, Singh V, Rustagi S, Chaudhary V (2025) Emergence of potassium solubilizing microbes-assisted crop processing for sustainable food production and microbial complexities. Food Bioprod Process
11. Dave S, Dave A, Radhakrishnan S, Das J, Dave S (2022) Biosensors for healthcare: an artificial intelligence approach. In: Biosensors for emerging and re-emerging infectious diseases. Elsevier, pp 365–383. https://doi.org/10.1016/B978-0-323-88464-8.00008-7
12. Do PC, Assefa YA, Batikawai SM, Reid SA (2023) Strengthening antimicrobial resistance surveillance systems: a scoping review. BMC Infect Dis 23(1):593. https://doi.org/10.1186/s12879-023-08585-2
13. Ekrami E, Pouresmaieli M, Shariati P, Mahmoudifard M (2021) A review on designing biosensors for the detection of trace metals. Appl Geochem 127:104902. https://doi.org/10.1016/j.apgeochem.2021.104902
14. Endale H, Mathewos M, Abdeta D (2023) Potential causes of spread of antimicrobial resistance and preventive measures in one health perspective – a review. Infect Drug Resist 16:7515–7545. https://doi.org/10.2147/IDR.S428837
15. Flynn CD, Chang D (2024) Artificial intelligence in point-of-care biosensing: challenges and opportunities. Diagnostics 14(11):1100. https://doi.org/10.3390/diagnostics14111100
16. Garzón V, Bustos RH, G. Pinacho D (2020) Personalized medicine for antibiotics: the role of nanobiosensors in therapeutic drug monitoring. J Personal Med 10(4):147. https://doi.org/10.3390/jpm10040147
17. Gopikrishnan M, Haryini S (2024) Emerging strategies and therapeutic innovations for combating drug resistance in Staphylococcus aureus strains: a comprehensive review. J Basic Microbiol 64(5):2300579. https://doi.org/10.1002/jobm.202300579
18. Gwenzi W, Musiyiwa K, Mangori L (2020) Sources, behaviour and health risks of antimicrobial resistance genes in wastewaters: a hotspot reservoir. J Environ Chem Eng 8(1):102220. https://doi.org/10.1016/j.jece.2018.02.028
19. Habeeb RAA, Nasaruddin F, Gani A, Hashem IAT, Ahmed E, Imran M (2019) Real-time big data processing for anomaly detection: a survey. Int J Inf Manag 45:289–307. https://doi.org/10.1016/j.ijinfomgt.2018.08.006
20. Haleem A, Javaid M, Singh RP, Suman R, Rab S (2021) Biosensors applications in medical field: a brief review. Sensors Int 2:100100. https://doi.org/10.1016/j.sintl.2021.100100
21. Heidt B, Siqueira WF, Eersels K, Diliën H, van Grinsven B, Fujiwara RT, Cleij TJ (2020) Point of care diagnostics in resource-limited settings: a review of the present and future of PoC in its most needed environment. Biosensors 10(10):133. https://doi.org/10.3390/bios10100133
22. Huang YP, Khabusi SP (2025) Artificial intelligence of things (AIoT) advances in aquaculture: a review. PRO 13(1):73. https://doi.org/10.3390/pr13010073
23. Khera HK, Mishra R (2024) Nucleic acid based testing (NABing): a game changer technology for public health. Mol Biotechnol 66(9):2168–2200. https://doi.org/10.1007/s12033-023-00870-4
24. Khorasani A, Moghim S, Wagemans J, Lavigne R, Mirzaei A (2024) Antibiotic profile classification of Proteus mirabilis using machine learning: an investigation into multidimensional radiomics features. Comput Biol Med 182:109131. https://doi.org/10.1016/j.compbiomed.2024.109131
25. Kunhikannan S, Thomas CJ, Franks AE, Mahadevaiah S, Kumar S, Petrovski S (2021) Environmental hotspots for antibiotic resistance genes. Microbiology 10(3):e1197. https://doi.org/10.1002/mbo3.1197
26. Kusi J, Ojewole CO, Ojewole AE, Nwi-Mozu I (2022) Antimicrobial resistance development pathways in surface waters and public health implications. Antibiotics 11(6):821. https://doi.org/10.3390/antibiotics11060821
27. Lee PI, Hsueh PR, Chuang JH, Liu MT (2024) Changing epidemic patterns of infectious diseases during and after COVID-19 pandemic in Taiwan. J Microbiol Immunol Infect. https://doi.org/10.1016/j.jmii.2024.07.002

28. Loosli K, Davis A, Muwonge A, Lembo T (2021) Addressing antimicrobial resistance by improving access and quality of care—a review of the literature from East Africa. PLoS Negl Trop Dis 15(7):e0009529. https://doi.org/10.1371/journal.pntd.0009529
29. Magnano San Lio R, Barchitta M, Maugeri A, La Rosa MC, Favara G, Agodi A (2023) Updates on developing and applying biosensors for the detection of microorganisms, antimicrobial resistance genes and antibiotics: a scoping review. Front Public Health 11:1240584. https://doi.org/10.3389/fpubh.2023.1240584
30. Majumder MAA, Rahman S, Cohall D, Bharatha A, Singh K, Haque M, Gittens-St Hilaire M (2020) Antimicrobial stewardship: fighting antimicrobial resistance and protecting global public health. Infect Drug Resist 13:4713–4738. https://doi.org/10.2147/IDR.S290835
31. Miller SA, Ferreira JP, LeJeune JT (2022) Antimicrobial use and resistance in plant agriculture: a one health perspective. Agriculture 12(2):289. https://doi.org/10.3390/agriculture12020289
32. Muteeb G, Rehman MT, Shahwan M, Aatif M (2023) Origin of antibiotics and antibiotic resistance, and their impacts on drug development: a narrative review. Pharmaceuticals 16(11):1615. https://doi.org/10.3390/ph16111615
33. Mutunga T, Sinanovic S, Harrison CS (2024) Integrating wireless remote sensing and sensors for monitoring pesticide pollution in surface and groundwater. Sensors 24(10):3191. https://doi.org/10.3390/s24103191
34. Nagraik R, Sharma A, Kumar D, Mukherjee S, Sen F, Kumar AP (2021) Amalgamation of biosensors and nanotechnology in disease diagnosis: mini-review. Sensors Int 2:100089. https://doi.org/10.1016/j.sintl.2021.100089
35. Neculai-Valeanu AS, Ariton AM, Radu C, Porosnicu I, Sanduleanu C, Amariţii G (2024) From herd health to public health: digital tools for combating antibiotic resistance in dairy farms. Antibiotics 13(7):634. https://doi.org/10.3390/antibiotics13070634
36. Pal A, Dubey SK, Goel S, Kalita PK (2024) Portable sensors in precision agriculture: assessing advances and challenges in soil nutrient determination. TrAC Trends Anal Chem 180:117981. https://doi.org/10.1016/j.trac.2024.117981
37. Pokharel S, Raut S, Adhikari B (2019) Tackling antimicrobial resistance in low-income and middle-income countries. BMJ Glob Health 4(6):e002104. https://doi.org/10.1136/bmjgh-2019-002104
38. Prickett M, Chambers T, Hales S (2024) When the first barrier fails: public health and policy implications of nitrate contamination of a municipal drinking water source in Aotearoa New Zealand. Australas J Water Res 28(1):64–73. https://doi.org/10.1080/13241583.2023.2272324
39. Ramesh M, Janani R, Deepa C, Rajeshkumar L (2022) Nanotechnology-enabled biosensors: a review of fundamentals, design principles, materials, and applications. Biosensors 13(1):40. https://doi.org/10.3390/bios13010040
40. Roberts W, McKee SA (2019) Mobile alcohol biosensors and pharmacotherapy development research. Alcohol 81:149–160. https://doi.org/10.1016/j.alcohol.2018.07.012
41. Rogdakis K, Psaltakis G, Fagas G, Quinn A, Martins R, Kymakis E (2024) Hybrid chips to enable a sustainable internet of things technology: opportunities and challenges. Discov Mater 4(1):4. https://doi.org/10.1007/s43939-024-00074-w
42. Rony MKK, Sharmi PD, Alamgir HM (2023) Addressing antimicrobial resistance in low and middle-income countries: overcoming challenges and implementing effective strategies. Environ Sci Pollut Res 30(45):101896–101902. https://doi.org/10.1007/s11356-023-29434-4
43. Sable H, Kumar V, Singh V, Rustagi S, Chaudhary V, Pandit S (2024) Nanosystems-enhanced electrochemical biosensors for precision in one health management. J Electrochem Soc 171(3):037527
44. Saxena S, Punjabi K, Ahamad N, Singh S, Bendale P, Banerjee R (2022) Nanotechnology approaches for rapid detection and theranostics of antimicrobial resistant bacterial infections. ACS Biomater Sci Eng 8(6):2232–2257. https://doi.org/10.1021/acsbiomaterials.1c01516
45. Shen Y, Anwar TB, Mulchandani A (2021) Current status, advances, challenges and perspectives on biosensors for COVID-19 diagnosis in resource-limited settings. Sensors Actuators Rep 3:100025. https://doi.org/10.1016/j.snr.2021.100025

46. Shrestha P, He S, Legido-Quigley H (2022) Antimicrobial resistance research collaborations in Asia: challenges and opportunities to equitable partnerships. Antibiotics 11(6):755. https://doi.org/10.3390/antibiotics11060755
47. Singh V, Kasana E, Batra J, Sable H, Saxena R (2022) Antimicrobial resistance: mechanisms, screening techniques and biosensors. J Pharm Negat Results 13:1724–1735
48. Struelens MJ, Ludden C, Werner G, Sintchenko V, Jokelainen P, Ip M (2024) Real-time genomic surveillance for enhanced control of infectious diseases and antimicrobial resistance. Front Sci 2:1298248. https://doi.org/10.3389/fsci.2024.1298248
49. Taha BA, Ahmed NM, Talreja RK, Haider AJ, Al Mashhadany Y, Al-Jubouri Q, Huddin AB, Mokhtar MHH, Rustagi S, Kaushik A (2024) Synergizing nanomaterials and artificial intelligence in advanced optical biosensors for precision antimicrobial resistance diagnosis. ACS Synth Biol 13(6):1600–1620
50. Uddin R, Koo I (2024) Real-time remote patient monitoring: a review of biosensors integrated with multi-hop IoT systems via cloud connectivity. Appl Sci 14(5):1876. https://doi.org/10.3390/app14051876
51. Upadhyay RG, Singh PK (2024) Strategies to combat drug resistance: innovations and challenges: A review. Biosci Biotechnol Res Asia 21(2):537. https://doi.org/10.13005/bbra/3245
52. Verma D, Singh KR, Yadav AK, Nayak V, Singh J, Solanki PR, Singh RP (2022) Internet of things (IoT) in nano-integrated wearable biosensor devices for healthcare applications. Biosens Bioelectron X 11:100153. https://doi.org/10.1016/j.biosx.2022.100153
53. Wei L, Zhu D, Cheng Q, Gao Z, Wang H, Qiu J (2024) Aptamer-based fluorescent DNA biosensor in antibiotics detection. Food Res Int 179:114005. https://doi.org/10.1016/j.foodres.2024.114005
54. Yi Z, Xu X, Meng X, Liu C, Zhou Q, Gong D, Zha Z (2023) Emerging markers for antimicrobial resistance monitoring. Chin Chem Lett 34(10):108238. https://doi.org/10.1016/j.cclet.2023.108238
55. Zhang Y, Hu Y, Jiang N, Yetisen AK (2023) Wearable artificial intelligence biosensor networks. Biosens Bioelectron 219:114825. https://doi.org/10.1016/j.bios.2022.114825

A Short Tutorial on Developing a Simple Biosensor for Antibiotic Abuse/Misuse

11

Nikhil Bhalla

11.1 Introduction

The increasing misuse and overuse of antibiotics in clinical, agricultural, and environmental settings have accelerated the emergence of antimicrobial resistance (AMR), posing a significant global health threat. Rapid and reliable detection of antibiotic residues is crucial for monitoring and mitigating this issue. Among various sensing technologies, colorimetric biosensors offer a simple, cost-effective, and user-friendly approach for antibiotic detection, making them ideal for point-of-care and field applications [1]. Refer to Table 11.1 for definitions of the terms misuse, overuse and abuse associated with antibiotics.

Colorimetric biosensors rely on visual changes in color to indicate the presence of antibiotics, eliminating the need for complex instrumentation. These sensors typically utilise plasmonic gold nanoparticles (AuNPs), enzyme-substrate reactions, or other nanomaterials that undergo distinct color transitions upon interaction with the target antibiotic. Such systems enable quick and intuitive detection, making them particularly useful in resource-limited settings, food safety monitoring, and clinical diagnostics.

This chapter provides a step-by-step guide to developing a simple colorimetric biosensor for detecting antibiotic residues. Associated key terms and definition are shared in Table 11.2. It covers key principles, material selection, fabrication methods, and performance evaluation techniques. By the end of this tutorial, readers will gain practical insights into designing a functional biosensor and its potential applications in combating antibiotic misuse.

N. Bhalla (✉)
Nanotechnology and Integrated Bioengineering Centre (NIBEC), School of Engineering, Ulster University, Belfast, Northern Ireland, UK
e-mail: n.bhalla@ulster.ac.uk

V. Chaudhary, N. Bhalla (eds.), *Biosensors for Tackling Antimicrobial Resistance (AMR)*, https://doi.org/10.1007/978-981-95-9151-0_11

Table 11.1 Antibiotic abuse/misuse/overuse

Term	Definition
Antibiotic misuse	Incorrect or inappropriate use of antibiotics, including using them for viral infections, incorrect dosing, or prematurely stopping a prescribed course
Antibiotic overuse	Excessive or unnecessary use of antibiotics, often as prophylaxis in agriculture or in clinical settings without clear indication of bacterial infection
Antibiotic abuse	Deliberate or habitual inappropriate use of antibiotics, such as self-medication without prescription or using leftover antibiotics from prior treatments

Table 11.2 Key terms and definitions for antibiotic colorimetric detection

Term	Definition
Antimicrobial Resistance (AMR)	The ability of microbes (e.g., bacteria, fungus, etc.) to survive exposure to drugs that would normally kill them.
Colorimetric Biosensor	A biosensor whose readout is a visible color change—simplest form of detection, often using plasmonic nanoparticles that shift color when they aggregate.
Gold Nanoparticles (AuNPs)	Nanoscale gold colloids (~10–100 nm) exhibiting strong localized surface plasmon resonance; their color and optical properties change upon aggregation.
Localized Surface Plasmon Resonance (LSPR)	Oscillation of conduction electrons in metal nanoparticles triggered by light, yielding intense absorbance peaks (e.g., red for dispersed AuNPs).
Turkevich Method	Classical chemical synthesis technique used for preparation of gold nanoparticles.
Aptamer	A short single-stranded DNA or RNA oligonucleotide that folds to bind a specific target molecule (e.g., an antibiotic) with high affinity and selectivity.
Aggregation	Process in which individual nanoparticles cluster to form larger structures due to attractive interactions between them.
UV–Vis Spectroscopy	An analytical technique that measures light absorbance vs. wavelength; used to monitor plasmon peaks (~520 nm for red AuNPs, ~650 nm when aggregated)
Calibration Curve	A graph showing relationship between known concentrations of the analyte and the measured sensor response, used to determine unknown concentration of analyte.
Point-of-Care Testing	Diagnostic testing performed at or near the site of patient care (or field), offering rapid, user-friendly results without the need for centralized labs.

11.2 Step-by-Step Protocol for Developing a Simple Colorimetric Biosensor for Antibiotic Detection

This protocol outlines a simple method for developing a gold nanoparticle (AuNP)-based colorimetric biosensor to detect antibiotic residues. The sensor changes color in response to the presence of antibiotics, providing a visual indication without requiring complex instruments.

11.2.1 Step 1: Understanding the Working Principle

Gold nanoparticles (AuNPs) exhibit unique optical properties due to localized surface plasmon resonances. In developing a colorimetric sensor we will utilize their red color (dispersed state) which changes to blue or purple (aggregated state) when interacting with antibiotics or other target molecules. This aggregation occurs due to charge interactions or specific binding events. Figure 11.1 shows a simple colorimetric detection of kanamycin which is based on target-induced AuNPs where these nanoparticles are functionalized with aptamer that trigger nanoparticle aggregation upon attachment of kanamycin [2].

11.2.2 Step 2: Materials and Chemicals Required

- **Gold chloride ($HAuCl_4$)**—for synthesizing AuNPs
- **Sodium citrate**—reducing agent for AuNPs formation
- **Antibiotic standard solutions** (In this tutorial, we have kanamycin)
- **Functional group specific to antibiotic** (Here we have an aptamer)
- **Buffer solutions** (PBS or Tris buffer)—to maintain pH stability
- **Glassware** (beakers, test tubes, micropipettes)
- **UV-Vis Spectrophotometer** (optional, for quantitative analysis)

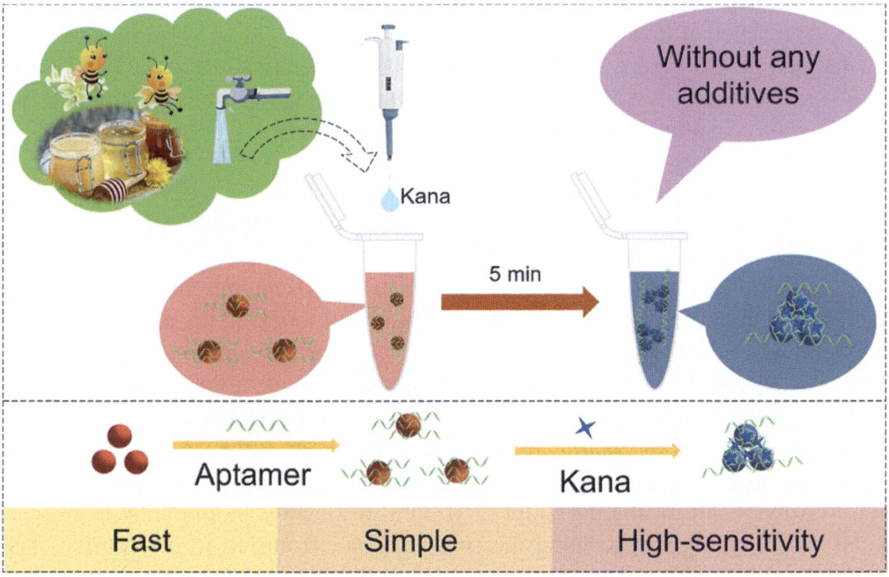

Fig. 11.1 Schematic showing colorimetric detection of kanamycin based on aggregation of aptamer-wrapped AuNPs. (This figure is reprinted with permission from [2])

11.2.3 Step 3: Synthesis of Gold Nanoparticles (AuNPs)

To synthesize AuNPs, dissolve 0.01 g of gold chloride ($HAuCl_4$) in 100 mL of distilled water in a beaker. Then heat (rapid boiling) 50 mL of the prepared solution to 100 °C before being injected with 2 mL of sodium citrate tribasic dihydrate, and a color change from yellow to black to dark red will be observed upon the formation of 20 nm diameter AuNPs. Allow the solution to cool to room temperature before use. More details on characteristics of these AuNPs synthesised using this method on can be found reference references discrinbing AuNP synthesis using Turkevich method [3, 4].

11.2.4 Step 4: Functionalization of AuNPs for Antibiotic Detection

Depending on the antibiotic type, we can use a suitable aptamer, antibody, or ligand that binds specifically to the target antibiotic. As mentioned earlier, in this tutorial we explain apatmer funcationalisation of AuNPs towards detection of kanamycin. The kanamycin aptamer used has a sequence of 5′-TGGGGGTTGAGGCTAAGCCG-3′ [2]. First a 5 μL aptamer (1.0 μM) was mixed with 40 μL AuNPs solution and incubated for 60 min at 37 °C to make aptamer coated AuNPs solution. To confirm the coating of AuNPs with the aptamer, UV-Vis spectrophotometer can be used to check the wavelength shifts in the LSPR spectrum of AuNPs which would confirm the binding of aptamer on AuNPs. One can also use other techniques like FTIR to confirm the presence of functional groups or SEM to observe the increase in the size of the nanoparticles. Figure 11.2 shows UV-Vis characterisation and SEM of the AuNPs in bare and funcationalised state alongside aggregation of nanoparticles when kanamycin attaches on the AuNPs (discussed later).

11.2.5 Step 5: Testing the Sensor for Antibiotic Detection

Once the aptamer coated AuNPs are ready, these AuNPs are introduced in the sample (usually in liquid form) consisting the target antibiotics. In the presence of specific antibiotics (here kanamycin) the AuNPs will aggregate and blue colour can be seen and depending on the concentration of the antiboitics the intensity of blue could change. Since we are focusing on the kanamycin detection, one can also test the developed sensor by creating different concentrations of the target kanamycin in a buffer solution (e.g., 0.1–10 μg/mL in PBS orTris), then adding the antibiotic solution to AuNPs and incubating to for 5–10 min. If kanamycin antibiotic is present, AuNPs will aggregate, changing the solution color from red to blue/purple. The intensity of the color change correlates with antibiotic concentration. Figure 11.3 shows the results related to colorimetric detection of kanamycin (named as Kana in the figure). We can also make a calibration curve of this response using a UV-Vis

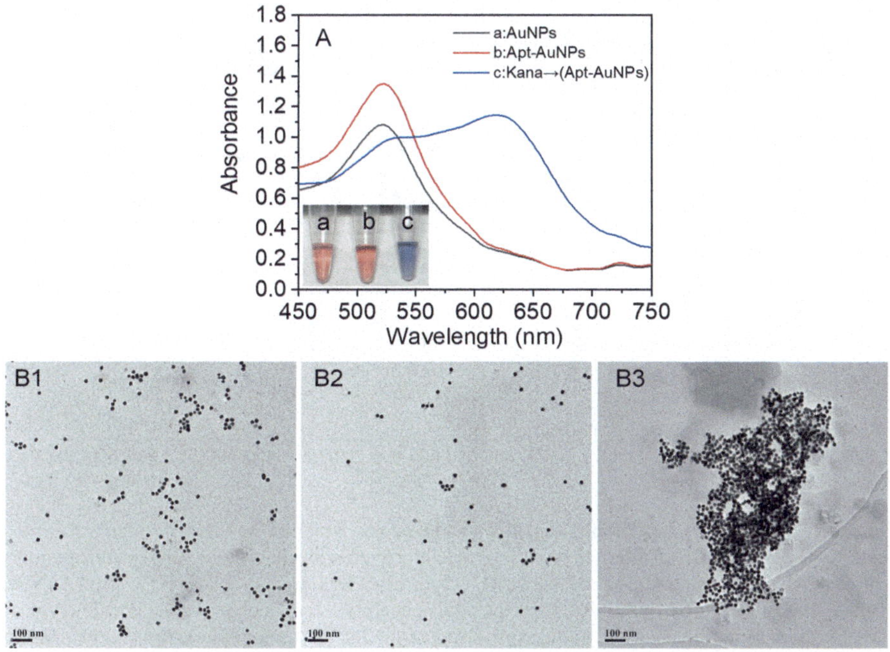

Fig. 11.2 (A) Typical UV–vis spectra and photographs of AuNPs (a), aptamer-wrapped AuNPs without (b) and with (c) kanamycin (the final concentration, 2.0 μM); (B) Typical TEM images of the AuNPs (13 nm)(B1), aptamer-wrapped AuNPs (B2), and aptamer-wrapped AuNPs in the presence of kanamycin (B3). (This figure is reprinted with permission from [2])

spectroscopy where either absorbance shifts or wavelength shifts can be plotted against the known concentration of the analyte. Please note that more advanced techniques such as Raman spectroscopy can also be integrated with this nanoparticle system to record and quantify the analyte binding response.

11.2.6 Step 6: Quantitative Analysis (Optional)

Qualitative testing can be performed visually, as a color change indicates the presence of antibiotics. For quantitative analysis, a UV-Vis spectrophotometer can measure absorbance in the range of 500–700 nm for dispersed AuNPs and around 650 nm for aggregated AuNPs. A standard calibration curve, plotting absorbance against antibiotic concentration, enables precise quantification. The naked eye provides a sufficient indication of antibiotic presence or absence (that is why we indicate that quantitative analysis is optional). However, the quantitative analysis would explicitly indicate the concentration antibiotics in the sample under test.

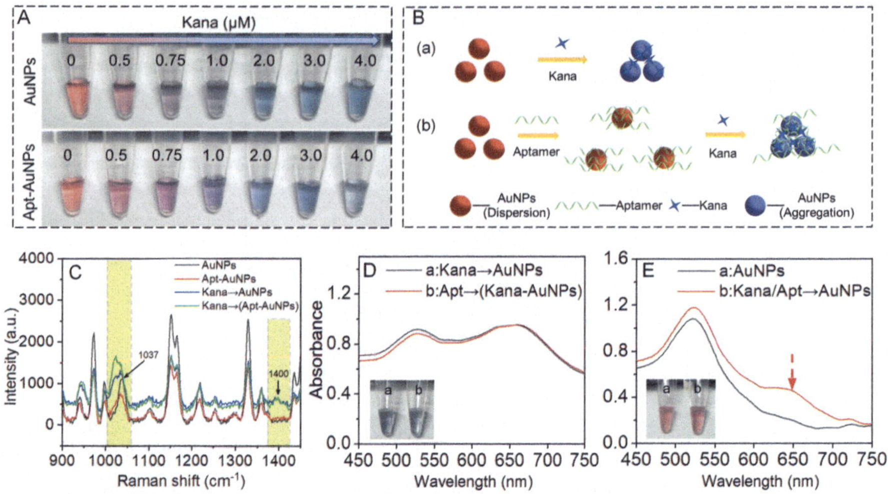

Fig. 11.3 (**A**) Typical photographs of AuNPs and aptamer-wrapped AuNPs with increasing concentrations of kana; (**B**) An alternative view of the colorimetric mechanism of AuNPs and aptamer-wrapped AuNPs with addition of kana; (**C**) Typical SERS spectra of AuNPs, Apt-AuNPs, Kana→AuNPs and Kana→(Apt-AuNPs) (the final concentration of kana was 2.0 μM); (**D**) Typical UV–vis spectra of Kana→AuNPs and Apt→(Kana-AuNPs) with the photographs shown in the insets; (**E**) Typical UV–vis spectra of AuNPs and Kana/Apt→AuNPs with the photographs shown in the insets. (This figure is reprinted with permission from [2])

11.2.7 Step 7: Validation and Field Testing (Optional)

Once the biosensor has been tested in the buffer solvents, it can be extended for tests in real-world samples (e.g., milk, water, blood serum) to evaluate its performance. A comparison table in different conditions can be compared included comparison with standard laboratory methods (e.g., HPLC, ELISA) for validation.

11.3 Use of Transduction Techniques Other Than Colorimetric Detection

While colorimetric methods are widely used due to their simplicity, several advanced transduction techniques offer higher sensitivity, selectivity, and real-time detection capabilities. These include electrochemical, optical, piezoelectric, Raman-based, fluorescence, thermal, magnetic, and mass spectrometry-based techniques [5–7].

11.3.1 Electrochemical Detection

Electrochemical biosensors are among the most sensitive techniques for detecting antibiotics. These sensors use electrodes to measure electrical signals generated by the interaction between antibiotics and biorecognition elements such as aptamers, enzymes, or antibodies. Techniques such as amperometry, voltammetry, and impedimetric sensing allow for low detection limits and rapid response times. For instance, an aptamer-based electrochemical biosensor can detect tetracycline with high specificity by monitoring changes in impedance when the antibiotic binds to the aptamer immobilized on an electrode [8].

11.3.2 Surface Plasmon Resonance (SPR) and Localized SPR (LSPR)

Optical biosensors utilizing SPR and LSPR techniques provide label-free and real-time detection of antibiotics. These methods rely on changes in the refractive index at the sensor surface when target molecules bind to a functionalized metal nanoparticle or thin metal film. LSPR, in particular, is highly sensitive due to the strong plasmonic effects at the nanoscale [9]. By designing multi-metallic LSPR biochips, antibiotic detection can be further optimized for multiplexing applications, enabling simultaneous detection of multiple antibiotics in complex samples using microfluidic based systems [10].

11.3.3 Piezoelectric and Acoustic Wave Biosensors

Piezoelectric sensors, including Quartz Crystal Microbalance (QCM) and Surface Acoustic Wave (SAW) sensors, operate based on mass-sensitive detection [11, 12]. When antibiotics bind to functionalized surfaces, they cause measurable frequency shifts, allowing label-free, real-time detection. SAW biosensors, in particular, offer high precision and can be integrated into portable devices for on-site antibiotic testing [13].

11.3.4 Surface-Enhanced Raman Scattering (SERS)

SERS-based biosensors amplify the Raman signal of antibiotic molecules using plasmonic nanostructures [14]. This technique enables ultra-sensitive, fingerprint-specific identification of antibiotics even at trace levels in food, water, and biological samples [15].

11.3.5 Fluorescence-Based Detection

Fluorescence biosensors employ fluorescent probes or quantum dots that emit light upon interacting with antibiotics [16]. Fluorescence resonance energy transfer (FRET)-based methods, for instance, can provide highly selective and sensitive detection by monitoring energy transfer between donor and acceptor fluorophores

[17]. These biosensors are widely used for rapid screening of antibiotic residues [18].

11.3.6 Thermal Biosensors (Calorimetric Detection)

Isothermal microcalorimetry detects heat changes associated with antibiotic interactions [19]. This label-free technique measures minute thermal variations that occur during biochemical reactions, making it useful for real-time monitoring of antibiotic presence in biological and clinical samples.

11.3.7 Magnetic Biosensors

Magnetic biosensors use magnetic nanoparticles functionalized with antibodies or aptamers to detect antibiotics [20]. By applying an external magnetic field, changes in the magnetic response can be measured, allowing for rapid and highly selective detection. Giant Magnetoresistance (GMR) sensors, for example, offer promising applications in point-of-care diagnostics [21].

11.3.8 Mass Spectrometry (MS) and Hybrid Techniques

Mass spectrometry (e.g., LC-MS, MALDI-TOF MS) [22] enables highly accurate detection and quantification of antibiotics in complex matrices. Combining MS with biosensor platforms enhances analytical performance, particularly for screening antibiotic residues in food and environmental samples.

11.4 Conclusions

In this tutorial, we have walked through the development of a simple, cost-effective colorimetric biosensor for rapid on-site antibiotic detection, using gold nanoparticles (AuNPs) as the sensing element. Starting from the Turkevich synthesis of monodisperse ~20 nm AuNPs, we demonstrated how to functionalize their surface with a kanamycin-specific aptamer, and how target-induced aggregation translates into a clear red-to-blue color change. We also showed how to characterize each step—with UV–Vis and TEM/SEM—and how to build a calibration curve for quantitative analysis.

Key Takeaways

- **Simplicity & accessibility:** All materials ($HAuCl_4$, citrate, aptamer) are commercially available, and no specialized instrumentation is required for detection—just the naked eye (or optional UV–Vis).

- **Specificity & sensitivity:** Aptamer functionalization confers high selectivity for kanamycin, and the aggregation-based readout yields detection down to low- nM levels.
- **Versatility:** The same workflow (synthesis → functionalization → colorimetric assay) can be adapted to other antibiotics by swapping in the appropriate aptamer or antibody.

Future Directions May Include

- **Matrix validation** in real-world samples (e.g., milk, serum, environmental waters), with minimal pretreatment.
- **Multiplexed formats**, using distinct nanoparticle sizes or labels to detect several antibiotics in parallel.
- **Integration with portable readers** (smartphone apps) for semi-quantitative field deployment.

By combining the optical simplicity of AuNP aggregation with the molecular precision of aptamer binding, this platform offers a powerful tool for combating antibiotic misuse and monitoring antimicrobial resistance at the point of need.

References

1. Aldewachi H, Chalati T, Woodroofe MN et al (2018) Gold nanoparticle-based colorimetric biosensors. Nanoscale 10(1):18–33
2. Ranran X, Cheng Y, Qi X et al (2022) Target-induced gold nanoparticles colorimetric sensing coupled with aptamer for rapid and high-sensitivity detecting kanamycin. Anal Chim Acta 1230:340377
3. Kimling J, Maier M, Okenve B et al (2006) Turkevich method for gold nanoparticle synthesis revisited. J Phys Chem B 110(32):15700–15707
4. Bradley Z, Bhalla N (2024) Combating prozone effects and predicting the dynamic range of naked-eye nanoplasmonic biosensors through capture bioentity optimization. ACS Measurement Science Au
5. Chaudhary V, Sable H, Bhadola P (2026) Harnessing complex light-matter interactions for point-of-care nano-optical biosensing. Adv Phys X 11(1):2609776
6. Chaudhary V, Bhadola P (2025) Artificial intelligence-powered nanosensor platforms for non-invasive breathomic diagnostics. Nanotechnol Sci Appl 18:611–641
7. Turner APF (2013) Biosensors: sense and sensibility. Chem Soc Rev 42(8):3184–3196
8. Jalalian SH, Karimabadi N, Ramezani M, Abnous K, Taghdisi SM (2018) Electrochemical and optical aptamer-based sensors for detection of tetracyclines. Trends Food Sci Technol 73:45–57
9. Bhalla N, Shen AQ (2024) Localized surface plasmon resonance sensing and its interplay with fluidics. Langmuir 40(19):9842–9854
10. Bhalla N, Lee D, Sathish S, Shen AQ (2017) Dual-mode refractive index and charge sensing to investigate complex surface chemistry on nanostructures. Nanoscale 9(2):547–554
11. Mandal D, Banerjee S (2022) Surface acoustic wave (SAW) sensors: physics, materials, and applications. Sensors 22(3):820

12. Haghdoust S, Arshad U, Mujahid A, Schranzhofer L, Lieberzeit PA (2021) Development of a MIP-based QCM sensor for selective detection of penicillins in aqueous media. Chemosensors 9(12):362
13. Kent CK, Ramakrishnan N, Kesuma HP (2024) Advancements in one-port surface acoustic wave (SAW) resonators for sensing applications: a review. IEEE Sensors J
14. Lee S, Dang H, Moon J-I et al (2024) SERS-based microdevices for use as in vitro diagnostic biosensors. Chem Soc Rev
15. Hong KY, Lima CD, de Albuquerque RJ, Poppi and Alexandre G Brolo. (2017) Determination of aqueous antibiotic solutions using SERS nanogratings. Anal Chim Acta 982:148–155
16. Lakshmi PR, Nanjan P, Kannan S, Shanmugaraju S (2021) Recent advances in luminescent metal-organic frameworks (LMOFs) based fluorescent sensors for antibiotics. Coord Chem Rev 435:213793
17. Zhou Y, Mahapatra C, Chen H et al (2020) Recent developments in fluorescent aptasensors for detection of antibiotics. Curr Opin Biomed Eng 13:16–24
18. Youn H, Lee K, Her J et al (2019) Aptasensor for multiplex detection of antibiotics based on FRET strategy combined with aptamer/graphene oxide complex. Sci Rep 9(1):7659
19. Christensen MH, Jakobsen TH, Lichtenberg M et al (2024) Antimicrobial susceptibility testing of bone and joint pathogens using isothermal microcalorimetry. APMIS 132(11):814–823
20. Cristea C, Tertis M, Galatus R (2017) Magnetic nanoparticles for antibiotics detection. Nano 7(6):119
21. Dey C, Yari P, Kai W (2023) Recent advances in magnetoresistance biosensors: a short review. Nano Futures 7(1):012002
22. Florio W, Baldeschi L, Rizzato C et al (2020) Detection of antibiotic-resistance by MALDI-TOF mass spectrometry: an expanding area. Front Cell Infect Microbiol 10:572909

The manufacturer's authorised representative in the EU is Springer Nature Customer Service Centre GmbH, Europaplatz 3, 69115 Heidelberg, Germany. If you have any concerns regarding our products, please contact ProductSafety@springernature.com

Printed and bound by CPI Group (UK) Ltd, Croydon, CR0 4YY
07/10/2026
02229349-0002